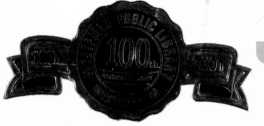

P9-DEI-112

THE FORCE PROGRAM

THE FORCE

PROGRAM

THE PROVEN WAY TO FIGHT CANCER THROUGH PHYSICAL ACTIVITY AND EXERCISE

JEFF BERMAN, FRAN FLEEGLER, M.D.,
AND JOHN HANC

BALLANTINE BOOKS • NEW YORK

This book is not intended as a substitute for medical advice. Consult your oncologist before beginning this program and follow the precautions and caveats that we have specified in every step of this program. Also, remember that the results of the FORCE program may vary, depending on the individual and the stage of the disease.

A Ballantine Book
Published by The Ballantine Publishing Group
Copyright © 2001 by Jeff Berman, Fran Fleegler, M.D., and John Hanc
Foreword copyright © 2001 by Karen Smyers

www.ballantinebooks.com

Library of Congress Cataloging-in-Publication Data
Berman, Jeff.
The FORCE program : the proven way to fight cancer through physical activity and exercise / Jeff Berman, Fran Fleegler, and John Hanc.—1st ed.
p.   cm.
1. Cancer—Exercise therapy.   2. Cancer—Physical therapy.   I. Fleegler, Fran.   II. Hanc, John.
III. Title.
RC271.P44 B47 2001
616.99'4062—dc21   2001035328

ISBN 0-345-44088-9

Manufactured in the United States of America

Designed by Ann Gold

First Edition: October 2001

10   9   8   7   6   5   4   3   2   1

CONTENTS

Acknowledgments   ix

Foreword by Karen Smyers   xi

INTRODUCTION

THE CASE FOR EXERCISE AND DIET IN THE FIGHT AGAINST CANCER   1

• A new paradigm in cancer treatment.

• The value of exercise, lifestyle, and stress management in cancer treatment.

CHAPTER ONE

HOW THE FORCE PROGRAM WAS BORN: JEFF BERMAN'S STORY   8

• The diagnosis of Jeff's cancer, his dramatic, successful battle against it, and
  how the FORCE program was developed out of his experience.

• What it has done for him and for others.

CHAPTER TWO

THE FORCE PROGRAM: WHAT WE DO, HOW IT WORKS   18

• Overview of FORCE, the country's most effective, comprehensive exercise-
  diet-stress management program for preventing and treating cancer.

• Getting yourself into the FORCE frame of mind.

CHAPTER THREE

GETTING STARTED   34

- Getting your doctor's permission—and giving yourself permission to embark on the FORCE program.
- Tips on getting started and sticking with it.

CHAPTER FOUR

STRESS MANAGEMENT   45

- Improve the quality of your day-to-day life; calm and center yourself with these mind-body techniques.

CHAPTER FIVE

EXERCISE AND PHYSICAL ACTIVITY   60

- Why physical exercise is at the heart of the FORCE program.
- Before you get started . . .
- Step-by-step through our three-stage activity/exercise program.
- Advice and specific instruction on each of the exercises.

CHAPTER SIX

NUTRITION   99

- The delicious, nutritious FORCE cancer-fighting diet.
- Guidelines, tips, important foods for fighting cancer.
- How to plan menus.
- Shopping and reading labels; surviving in restaurants.
- Supplements and herbs: What's the story?

CHAPTER SEVEN

EXERCISE AND MOVEMENT REGIMENS FOR SPECIFIC CANCERS   125

- How to tailor the FORCE program depending on your cancer site: breast, prostate, lung, lymphoma, leukemia, brain, and colorectal cancers.

CHAPTER EIGHT

THE K-FORCE PROGRAM FOR CHILDREN   149

- Overview of the K-FORCE program for children with cancer, and how
  the program developed.
- Ways to get kids relaxed, to get them moving and, believe it or not,
  to get them eating a healthier diet.

Afterword by Jeff Berman, FORCE Program Founder   166

Resources   169

Index   179

ACKNOWLEDGMENTS

The authors would like to thank the following people for helping make the FORCE program, and this book, a reality.

For their invaluable help on this book, we thank veteran wordsmith Mark Will-Weber for his contributions to the manuscript, Mike Mathis for his illustrations, and Mike's former teacher Peter Voci for what turned out to be an accurate recommendation of his ex-student's talent and affable personality. Thank you to Dr. Steve Jonas for bringing this whole team together; our agent, Linda Konner, for her wise counsel; our editor, Leslie Meredith, and her assistant, Abby Durden.

Special thanks to the FORCE advisory board, particularly three members who gave so much of their time and expertise to this project: Heather Salomon, MS, RD; John Buzzerio, MS; and Bette Jean Rosenhagen, CSW.

We also thank these members of the advisory board for their important contributions to this book and to the FORCE program: Genevieve Lowry, CSW; Regina Grieco, ACE; Juel Bedford, ACE; Kathy Sutherland, ACE; Douglas Kalman, MS, RD; Kathryn Kash, Ph.D.; Deborah Kennedy, MS; Elena Ladas, RD; Frank Sheridan, MS; and Karrie Zampini, CSW.

Jeff Berman would like to thank Fred Lebow, founder of the New York City Marathon, for seeing in me what I didn't see in myself; all the cancer patients who've entrusted me and taught me about life; the Greater New York City Affiliate of The Susan G. Koman Breast Cancer Foundation, Inc. and Harlem YMCA for funding the FORCE vision and helping to bring it to the women of Harlem; and Gerald Schiller at the National Executive Service Corps., who advised me to write this book. Also, thanks to Les Winter of the Achilles Track Club; W. H. Ju, Ph.D., a guide and teacher; Ingrid Vai for her gentle way and for being there in the good times and bad; and my special canine pals, Irv and Tango, who are always with me.

John Hanc would like to thank colleagues at *Newsday* and the New York Institute of Technology, specifically, editors Phyllis Singer for her encouragement, Barbara Schuler for her interest, and Bob Henn for his good cheer, and Dr. Edward Guiliano, Dr. Robert Vogt, and Professor James Fauvell for their willingness to make accommodations in my teaching schedule, enabling me to deliver this manuscript. And, of course, a special thanks to my immediate family—wife, Donna; son, Andrew; mom, Dolores; and father-in-law, George—for their unwavering love and support—and to all my friends, colleagues, and training partners for their encouragement and companionship.

Dr. Fran Fleegler: Energy, inspiration, and passion for these ideas were made possible by my home team (Ed, Aryn, Ethan, and Sara) as well as my athletic and my "professional" teams. I am forever grateful for support, partnership, courage, and for all of the hugs along the way.

FOREWORD

Karen Smyers

Women's Winner, 1995 Hawaii Ironman Triathlon World Championship; seventh-place finisher, 2000 U.S. Women's Olympic Triathlon Trials; thyroid cancer survivor

As a professional triathlete who makes a living from having a fit and healthy body, I was shocked beyond belief when the ultrasound indicated a high probability of thyroid cancer. I thought that cancer was something that happened to other people, certainly not a professional triathlete. Certainly not someone who trained twenty hours a week. Certainly not someone capable of completing an Ironman distance triathlon—that's a 2.4-mile swim, 112-mile bike ride, and 26.2-mile marathon run, done in succession in a time of nine hours . . . and in the heat of Hawaii, yet!

But that someone with cancer was me. When the biopsy confirmed the cancer, I was forced to confront my worst fears. The body I had relied on, the hard-earned fitness that had enabled me to earn a living, now seemed to be letting me down. Being both a cancer victim and a professional athlete was so incongruous that at first I had a hard time accepting it. My notion of a cancer victim was of someone sickly, pale, inactive, and bedridden.

At first, I tried to figure out ways the diagnosis could have been a mistake.

My mother has had an enlarged thyroid for a decade, so maybe I had inherited that and there was really nothing to worry about! Or perhaps they mixed up my biopsy sample with that woman in the waiting room, the one who had a large protrusion sticking out of her neck. Of course! Hers had probably come up negative, because it was really mine!

When I eventually ran out of viable theories, I began to accept my diagnosis. The first change I made in thinking about having cancer was striking the word "victim" from my vocabulary. I started thinking instead about being a cancer *survivor*. Although that may sound like simply a matter of semantics, it also represents a change in attitude: I couldn't change the fact that I had cancer, but I certainly could control the way I would deal with it. And that is what I decided to focus on.

One way I would deal with it was to make sure that my sense of humor remained intact. I made jokes about my ensuing treatment, that one of the benefits of receiving radioactive iodine would be that I would be able to run at night without wearing reflective clothing. (It didn't matter to me if anyone else thought it was funny, as long as I did.)

I had surgery to remove the thyroid in December 1999 while I was also recovering from a broken collarbone from the last race of the season. (When it rains, it pours, right?) My husband and I decided there was no reason not to continue to chase my dream of making the first U.S. Olympic Team in triathlon, a sport that made its Olympic debut in the 2000 Games in Sydney, Australia. The trials would be held in May, which gave me four months to recover from the surgery and the collarbone injury. It would be a long shot, I realized, but I knew I would regret not trying more than I would regret not making the team.

As I pursued my athletic goals, as I got back into the groove of my training, my faith in my body was gradually restored. I was reenergized by the immediacy and importance of the goal I had chosen. I had no time for self-pity, but plenty of time for treating my body well and egging it on to be the best it could be. I was soon doing workouts that were comparable to the best workouts I had ever done—precancer, premotherhood, and all.

When the trials date finally approached, I found myself just being happy to make it to the starting line healthy. Though I finished seventh in the race—not good enough to make the Olympic Team—I felt great, and I was totally at peace with my effort.

After some reflection on the race and its outcome, I realized that the quest to make the Olympic Team was one of the most therapeutic and rewarding experiences I could have undertaken after the discovery of my thyroid cancer. My husband and I had sailed through the surgery and emotional trauma because of the confidence that exercise restored in me about my physical self. This physical boost can be achieved by anyone battling cancer, not just professional athletes. The sense of well-being that comes with regular exercise and good nutrition is attainable by anyone who is motivated enough to try. Whether it's walking a few minutes a day or running marathons like Jeff Berman, the founder of the FORCE program and a coauthor of this book, the sense of regaining some control over your body can bring amazing results and vast improvements in your quality of life.

Unfortunately, the medical establishment doesn't have time to counsel and encourage cancer patients to exercise. From my experience, doctors have their hands full just fitting in quick consults about the disease itself around their busy surgery schedules. Their expertise is confined to their specialties and they generally don't have the time or inclination to look at the whole-body approach to fighting the disease.

That is why I believe the FORCE program is so valuable. Until now, this unique exercise/nutrition/stress management program for cancer patients was available only to people in the New York City area. Now, through this book, it's available to you. This is not designed to replace your doctor's care, but to augment it. It's a way to improve your condition and your life, a way that is within *your* control. And it doesn't rely on surgery or radiation or a pill, but on your own resolve, your own efforts.

It is one of the most important steps you can take in going from cancer victim to cancer survivor. Good luck!

THE CASE FOR EXERCISE AND DIET IN THE FIGHT AGAINST CANCER

Twenty or thirty years ago, a person who had a heart attack and survived was told not to take the stairs, not to have arguments, not to get too excited, not even to have sex for so many days or weeks. They were called "cardiac cripples."

Well, there are no more cardiac cripples today. But physicians, friends, family, and society are doing the same thing with cancer patients. We are crippling them.

Cardiologists no longer tell their patients to sit still and take it easy. Within weeks or even days of leaving the hospital, most heart patients are walking on treadmills or pedaling stationary bicycles under the supervision of cardiac rehab specialists. They are urged to modify their diet and increase their physical activities.

Not so cancer patients. The medical literature their doctors refer to is full of warnings not to do this, not to do that. In one of the standard oncology texts, a nine-hundred-page tome, there are only *three* vague paragraphs about exercise.

Odd, isn't it? Most public health organizations acknowledge the role exercise plays in helping protect against certain forms of cancer (particularly those of the breast and bowel). A widely publicized report from the Harvard School of Public Health in 1997 estimated that 65 percent of cancer deaths are caused by unhealthy lifestyles and are thus preventable. The authors of the Harvard study cited smoking cessation, proper diet, and daily exercise as the best means of reducing the risk of developing a number of types of cancer.

If physical activity and lifestyle can play a role in preventing cancer, couldn't they play a role in treatment? You would think this question would inspire at least some interest among researchers. But mainstream medicine has all but ignored the relationship between exercise and cancer treatment. Only one of fourteen thousand investigations listed last year with the National Cancer Institute, for example, dealt with exercise. As Dr. Fran Fleegler, one of the coauthors of this book, notes, "There are no guidelines, no protocols for exercise. But that's what we physicians and health care providers should be doing with our patients: trying to get them to move and strengthen their muscles."

That's exactly what the FORCE program does.

FORCE, an acronym for Focus on Rehabilitation and Cancer Education, helps individuals find the best activities to boost the effectiveness of their medical treatments and, in tandem with dietary modifications and stress management techniques, helps them heal. The FORCE program is a plan for living and dealing optimistically and actively with cancer.

You'll notice that we have not said anything here about "cures." We are not suggesting that exercise, nutrition, and stress management will cure your cancer. But the goal of any treatment plan is curative or palliative in nature, meaning that the treatment attempts to eliminate the disease or to alleviate the effects of the disease and maintain the patient's level of comfort. It's important to clarify from the outset the expected goals of any treatment, and what the goals of this book and our FORCE program really are.

For example, Stage IV metastatic cancer is incurable. No amount of exercise, diet, or stress management—or chemo and radiation, for that matter—will change that. But that doesn't mean that there's nothing we can do except await an inevitable demise. One can convert incurable cancer into a chronic condition that requires continual treatment. Even though the cancer will never be totally gone, it will be absolutely and totally manageable. (And if that sounds terrible, consider this: diabetes, hypertension, and hepatitis are long-term illnesses that are not curable but are manageable. People live long lives with these illnesses, just as they do with many forms of cancer.)

The experiences of Dr. Fleegler, Jeff Berman, and the FORCE program prove this. There are hundreds of men and women today—patients, graduates of the FORCE program—who are living happy, full lives. The medicine that their doctors gave them had something to do with their survival, sure. So did luck. But don't let anyone tell you that what they did for themselves didn't matter. Their lifestyle—what they ate, how they exercised, and how they managed stress—were all vital components in their successful recoveries.

THE LIFESTYLE APPROACH TO CANCER REHAB: EVIDENCE MOUNTS

Dr. Fleegler will admit something that many of her colleagues might not: There is a lot about her specialty, oncology, that is still not well understood. The knowledge base is changing constantly. Oncology is a young medical specialty, and scientific research is daily uncovering more about the underlying mechanisms of cancer. There are exciting, promising developments going on in labs and clinics all over the country. Understanding molecular mutations and genetic codes may help the next generation or next year's potential cancer patients. Yet, we must be honest: It may not be able to help you.

But we know something that can.

Most of the heavily funded cancer research is looking at genetics or at the effectiveness of various drug and chemotherapy combinations. Yet, a spate of new studies has studied exercise and lifestyle and their relationship to cancer—with interesting results. Most of these studies have been published not in the primary oncological publications, but in sports medicine journals. Most of them have been conducted not by M.D.s but by Ph.D.s, cancer care providers, and exercise physiologists. The buzz surrounding this burgeoning new area of health care literature is exciting. Because what these researchers have found seems to suggest that what Dr. Fleegler and others have suspected is right: People can fight cancer more effectively when exercise, good nutrition, and stress management are added to their medical treatments.

One of the most important of these studies was conducted in 1999 among cancer patients in a health club in Santa Barbara, California. The subjects, people who suffered from various types of cancers, were put on a program of aerobic exercise, weight training, and flexibility-relaxation techniques. After ten weeks, subjects showed a 43 percent increase in strength and more than doubled their time spent on aerobic exercise machines. In addition, they reported significant improvement in their day-to-day lives: they said that they were better able to participate in recreational and leisure activities in addition to routine household chores. The patients also reported that they had a markedly lower perception of pain.

The program used for this study is now being marketed to health clubs, and the researchers hope to develop a nationwide certification program for trainers. That's a positive step, but it won't help the millions of Americans with cancer who don't have access to the kind of first-rate facility that has such a program. Nor will it be of much value to those who are intimidated by gyms or too sick to leave their home. But the FORCE program will help all these people.

The FORCE program is about using movement and exercise to help you heal—even if you weren't active prior to your diagnosis, even if you've never been to a gym. We're not talking about running marathons, cycling the Tour de France, or lifting huge amounts of weight. What we want you to do—at least to begin with—are simple, everyday activities: climb stairs, carry the groceries, walk to the mailbox. Even such moderate levels of exercise are beneficial. They will help speed your recovery, if not from the disease itself, from the chemotherapy and radiation treatments, the "cures" that sometimes seem worse than the problem.

Your medical treatments are important. But so are the things that you do—or, in some cases, don't do enough—in your daily life: exercise, eat well, and practice stress management techniques that can strengthen the body and the mind. Even if your doctor overlooks these factors in your cancer-fighting treatments, you can explore them on your own—with the help of this book.

Until recently, the mainstream medical community has ignored both the anecdotal and the growing scientific evidence that suggests that physically fit cancer patients (a concept, by the way, that is not a contradiction in terms) can fight the disease better, can improve their quality of life, and may even live longer.

The majority of doctors may not be interested in this evidence, but 1.4 million American cancer patients and their families are. Presumably, you're one of them. If so, we want to tell you that this is a program and a book of hope. Again, we are not saying that exercise, diet, and other lifestyle modifications are a cure for cancer. But they can help cancer patients feel stronger mentally as well as physically. That may be the primary lesson we can learn from Lance Armstrong, the man who came back from cancer to win the Tour de France, generally regarded as the world's toughest endurance event, twice.

FORCE: THE PROVEN LIFESTYLE PROGRAM TO HELP FIGHT CANCER

No one was rooting harder for Lance Armstrong than Jeff Berman.

Although Jeff has never met the two-time Tour de France winner and best-selling author, he has worked with a number of Olympians, including wrestler

Jeff Blatnick, marathoner Mark Conover, and track star Marty Liquori, all of whom had cancer. Perhaps better than most, Berman could understand what Armstrong had been through and the true magnitude of his achievement.

Berman, now forty-three, was preparing for a triathlon in 1990 when he discovered a lump in his neck. Tests revealed that he had chronic lymphocytic leukemia, a form of cancer. He was told that it was manageable, but not curable—and that there really was nothing that could be done for him until he got sick.

An athlete since high school, Berman, a native of Spring Valley, New York, decided to do what came naturally: he kept moving, kept training, kept competing. But in 1993, he got sick. The disease struck his lymph nodes, causing them to thicken, which affected his breathing. He was preparing for the New York City Marathon at the time and managed to complete his training and finish the race.

Eight years later, Jeff is still running marathons. But now he also runs the FORCE program, which he founded as a direct result of his own experience as a cancer patient. Today, patients are referred to Berman from the major New York–area cancer centers—world-renowned hospitals, including the Post-Treatment Resource Program at Memorial Sloan-Kettering, New York University Medical Center, Columbia Presbyterian, and Beth Israel. Why? Because professionals at these hospitals know that the program works. They know that FORCE is one of only a handful of such programs in the country. And unlike some of the other hospital-based lifestyle programs, the FORCE program can be followed by people at home.

This book will show you how to fight the disease by strengthening your body; how exercise, proper diet, and stress management can give you the physical and psychological edge that can make all the difference; how simple activities can help repair the damage of chemo and restore your own sense of self and well-being. This book will show you that there is good reason to hope, that there are things you can do to help yourself, in real and tangible ways. We'll show you the way, and we'll start by telling you Jeff Berman's story. In his own way, he's as inspirational as Lance Armstrong, because though few can personally relate to a world-class athlete, anyone—certainly anyone with cancer—can identify with the feelings of a regular guy who one day finds a lump in his neck and, in that instant, knows the rest of his life will never be the same.

CHAPTER ONE

HOW THE FORCE PROGRAM WAS BORN: JEFF BERMAN'S STORY

At the beginning of 1990, Jeff Berman's life was almost perfect.

He had been married since 1987, became a homeowner the following year, was a rising star in the lucrative TV ad sales business in Manhattan, and commuted home to suburban Bridgewater, New Jersey, every night. Life was good and looked as if it was going to get even better. Berman was, in his own words, "ready to fly."

But his flight was rerouted, as he explains.

"Sometime in February, something in my neck just felt wrong. It was swollen in one spot. I figured I'd give it a few weeks and it would go away. But after three weeks, I could still feel it. So I had my doctor take a look at it. He said it was probably nothing, and to give it a few more weeks. I asked him, 'You think it's a problem?' And he said, 'Nah, you've got a million-to-one shot of this being a problem.'"

Those sounded like good odds. So Berman went back to his day-to-day life, which included sports. A wrestler in high school, Berman had maintained a similar fitness regimen as an adult. He lifted weights three or four times a week and, a few years earlier, had started running and cycling. He was planning to do his first triathlon—the swim, bike, run event—in April.

Three weeks after his first visit, Berman returned to the doctor. The lump on his neck was bigger and longer. This time the doctor ordered tests: chest X rays, blood tests, and more. Everything came up normal. The one test left that they needed to do was a biopsy.

"I go in for this biopsy, and I'm sitting in the hospital, in one of these gowns they give you. There's a guy next to me in a wheelchair. I remember he started telling me how the same thing happened to him. It was a 'Let's just do a precautionary test,' and the next thing he knows, he's got lung cancer and they're operating on him. I remember listening to him sympathetically, but it still never clicked that the same thing could happen to me. In fact, I was so relaxed that when I went in for the biopsy and lay down on the operating table, I fell asleep."

The weekend after the biopsy, Berman completed his triathlon. Two weeks went by, and he was back into his normal routine, when his physician called. "We need to talk," he said. "What's the matter?" Berman replied. "Just come in," said the doctor. Berman arrived at the doctor's office between sales calls. He had his briefcase in hand and his three-piece suit on.

"I was brought into his office, and there he is—Dr. Newman, a great guy— with his head in his hands. I thought, 'Oh, shit, the million-to-one shot came through.' "

Newman looked up at Berman and gave him the bad news. He had chronic lymphocytic leukemia, a disease that primarily strikes people over sixty-five. Berman was told to seek out the help of specialists. The first one he went to, an eminent oncologist in Manhattan, told him that there was nothing that could be done for him until he developed symptoms. In other words, he had to get sick before he could be treated for the cancer that was already there. The next special- ist, Dr. Bruce Raphael at New York University, told him something a little differ- ent. He said that Berman was the youngest patient he'd ever met with the disease and that the best thing to do was to track it and retest it every six months. Other than that: Go back to leading your life.

"I left his office thinking that now I had a guy to work with. Now I had a plan. I kept training, I kept working, I felt good."

At the urging of his primary physician, Berman went to see another specialist, a noted oncologist at Memorial Sloan-Kettering Cancer Center. So noted, in fact, that Berman had to wait four and a half hours to see him. And he told him the same thing as the first specialist: Yes, you have this disease; no, there's nothing that can be done for you now.

"So I figure since I waited half a day to see this Dr. Big Shot, I better ask him a couple of questions, and one of them was about my training. I said, 'Doc, I'm lifting weights, I'm running, I'm cycling, I'm training for my second triathlon. Won't that help me?' And I'll never forget the way he looked at me. Like I was a fool. 'Oh yeah,' he said. 'You probably won't die of a heart attack.' Then he paused like that was his punch line. 'But it won't have anything to do with your cancer. It's going to progress until you get sick and you'll need chemotherapy or a bone marrow transplant or you'll die.'"

Berman stormed out of the office.

"I wanted to pummel that guy. I was not angry about the disease. I was not shocked or dismayed. I didn't think I was going to die. But I was angry with him. Angry at the way he dismissed me, angry at his arrogance, angry that I was, to him, just another line on a predictable graph. Since then, I've heard similar stories from other cancer patients about other doctors. Some of them may be good at treating cancer, but they're no good at treating people."

Berman finally threw in his hat with the oncologist at NYU. Bruce Raphael, M.D., had impressed him with his honesty and his sense of humor—and the fact that he was willing to develop a plan to monitor the disease: blood tests every three months, CT scans and bone marrow biopsies every six months. The first bone marrow biopsy was also Berman's first clue that maybe his lifestyle was a factor in his favor.

"The way they explained the bone marrow biopsy to me was: Think of the patient as a bottle of fine wine. They've got to stick a corkscrew into you deep enough to get a taste of what's inside. So I'm on the table, and Raphael is trying to do this, using this long needle that they can push all the way down into the bone until they strike marrow. And soon, he's sweating, he's grunting and groaning. And I'm giggling. Giggling despite the fact that this is the most indescribable pain I've ever felt. The anesthetic doesn't help, because they're going six inches deep into your body. But I was still laughing. Because, as Raphael later told me, my bones were like steel from years of weight training."

Between the laughter and the tears, Berman got a flash of insight: "For the first time, I realized that maybe my strength, my conditioning could be an asset."

That strength would be put to the test in other ways. A few days after the bone marrow biopsy, Berman and his wife met, as they usually did, at the PATH station near their home in New Jersey after commuting from a day's work in the city. They stopped to pick up pizza at a little place in the station they frequented. They got into their car, and were preparing to drive home. Suddenly:

"I just started to cry. I don't know where it came from. The floodgates opened. It was because for the first time, I had stopped thinking about the future. I was, as they say, 'living in that moment.' And I guess, quite frankly, it all caught up with me. I felt better afterward, but I haven't cried about the disease since. My approach to the cancer began to crystallize in my mind. I had now accepted the reality of it, but at the same time, I had formulated my plan. I decided I was going to beat up on the disease before it beat up on me. And the way I was going to do that was by always looking forward, always looking to the next step, and always doing something to improve my health, improve my body, and improve my mental condition. I intended to stay one step ahead of the damn disease."

Some people talk about fighting cancer with optimism, with cheer, with laughter. Berman, being naturally a cheerful and good-humored guy, did that and something more: he decided to fight it by taking further action. He had already spent nearly $50,000 on medical visits, so he began to spend time trying to gather information about the disease, about cancer support, cancer services, cancer treatment. He was disappointed in what was available. All he got from the established cancer foundations and organizations were brochures and talk about "loss" and "bereavement."

"Loss, loss, loss. That's all I kept reading, all I kept hearing about. I never for an instant thought about my disease as a 'lose' proposition. I always thought in terms of How do we get over this? Where can I get more information? Who can help me? What actions can I take?"

One of the actions was not pleasant, but it was necessary.

"I realized that although I'd been married for five years, I didn't have a partner. I didn't have somebody who understood what was happening or what I was trying to do. She smoked and she continued to smoke after my diagnosis. That caused friction. We tried to get on the same page in terms of diet and trying to exercise and helping me attack the disease. But it never seemed to work. I realized that I had to make a change."

The couple separated and, in September 1992, Berman and his wife divorced. Things got complicated for a while. Jeff even had to declare bankruptcy. Eventually, he found an apartment in Manhattan and a new job. For a year, he forgot about his cancer and focused on rebuilding his life. But one night in October 1993, he woke up to the sound of his own breathing—a prolonged wheeze every time he inhaled. The disease had come alive and attacked the lymph nodes that surround the neck and throat. Raphael told him it was time for chemo. A month after finishing the 1994 NYC Marathon, Berman began six months of chemotherapy.

"I remember saying to myself, 'You better be prepared for your life to become a mess. Your hair's going to fall out. You're going to feel weak. You're going to get sick.' This is what I thought, because this is what I had been told."

He had been told wrong. Berman didn't get sick, didn't lose his hair, didn't even feel too weak. Was it his fitness? Was it his careful attention to his exercise, to his diet, to his attitude? Or was it, as some would say, just luck? Five years later, the growing number of studies on exercise and cancer treatment would seem to suggest that it wasn't just Berman's good fortune, but his good health and fitness that enabled him to keep feeling good during chemo.

On a December morning during his chemotherapy, Jeff took a run in Central Park, where he spotted a thin man with a goatee, Fred Lebow. One of the men behind the running boom of the 1970s, Lebow was a Romanian emigrant who spoke with a thick accent. He had worked in the garment industry for years before taking up jogging. In the late 1960s, he got involved with the fledgling New York Road Runners Club, then a tiny organization generally viewed as a few nuts running around in the equivalent of underwear. But Lebow's vision, creativity, and passion for his new sport transformed the club into a growing, healthy, and trendy organization. In September 1970, he organized the first New York City Marathon in Central Park. Fifty-five runners finished that day. Six years later, Lebow had managed to persuade the city to run the race through the five boroughs. By the end of the 1980s, the NYC Marathon was the world's largest 26.2-miler, with nearly thirty thousand finishers, and was well known as one of the world's great sports spectacles. "Fred was the man. Fred was the guy everybody in the running community knew and looked up to," says Berman.

But in February 1990, Lebow had been diagnosed with brain cancer. During a presentation at the club's annual awards dinner, he confused two people he knew well: then–*New York Post* writer Dave Hanson and *Newsday*'s John Hanc, one of the coauthors of this book. Lebow's brain cancer was serious. And yet, he too fought back. And in November 1992, in a memorable and nationally televised display of courage and perseverance, Lebow ran the New York City Marathon. Accompanied by friends and reporters (including coauthor Hanc), he went the distance through a city that probably would have elected him mayor that day. There were cheers, tears, hugs, headlines, and, everywhere, crowds of people applauding his effort, awed by his achievement.

It was a year later that Berman spotted Lebow in the park.

"I was coming one way, he was going the other. He didn't look at me. I kept going and then stopped. I'm not sure why, but I felt that we had something in common. We were both fighting cancer, and I felt there was something I needed to do. I ran back and stopped him. When I told him I had cancer, he immediately became very warm. Cancer will do that to you. You change, you feel empathy and a bond with people that you never felt before."

Right there in Central Park, Berman the salesman pitched Lebow on an idea that would eventually become the FORCE program. It was a spur-of-the-moment proposal.

"I told Fred, 'You know, it's great that you brought this idea front and center, the idea that you can get cancer and survive and keep going and run a marathon. But I think there's more we can do, especially through the Road Runners Club. You and I are not the only people involved with running in New York who have cancer.' "

Berman later admitted that he wasn't really sure what he had in mind. Just something "to bring people together." But Lebow saw something in Berman and invited him over to his office to discuss the idea. They met in the stately old brownstone on East 89th Street that serves as the New York Road Runners Club headquarters.

"We sat down, and Lebow said, 'Would you like to start a support group?' I said, 'Yes.' He looked at me and said, 'Do you know how we start?' Before I could say anything, he said, 'We start by starting.' "

And that's what started it. An ad in the club's magazine, some calls and flyers posted around the club. On March 9, 1994, the first meeting of the New York

Road Runners Club's Cancer Support Group was held in a conference room at the old brownstone. Ten runners and walkers joined Berman and Lebow for a freewheeling discussion about cancer and running. But it wasn't the kind of discussion Berman was used to hearing at other cancer groups and among other cancer patients.

"It wasn't about fear. It wasn't about dying. It was about living! That was what was so amazing."

Berman found himself falling into the role of group facilitator. The discussions—and they were just discussions at that point—left him, and everyone else, feeling energized, upbeat, optimistic. And then they would all go out for a run or a walk through the park and feel even better.

"I was going through chemo this whole time and here I was telling people what they could do to change their lives, improve their fitness, and feel better. I came home one night and I said to my girlfriend, 'You know, I think I finally found a way to stay alive.' "

That fall, Berman filed for not-for-profit status. He called his new corporation Cancer Support Services. "We really became an organization at that point! It was so satisfying. It had become more than an idea, more than an experiment." This was real support, hope made concrete, healing made possible.

In addition to the weekly meetings, Berman began to fine-tune the principles that would become the core of his approach to dealing with the disease. The first was the value of exercise. The second was nutrition: he was eating more carefully, emphasizing a higher-carb, low-fat diet of vegetables, fruits, and whole grains. The third element of what would eventually become the FORCE program presented itself in April 1994, when Berman attended a meeting of an organization called Friends in Deed and learned about the power of relaxation.

A support group for people with all kinds of illnesses, primarily HIV-related, the meeting started with a moderator saying, "Okay, everybody, hold hands." For ten minutes, the group sat quietly, meditating. It was Berman's first and unexpected experience with the use of relaxation techniques to help cope with serious illness.

"I realized this was something really special. For two hours afterward, I listened intently and scribbled down notes as people discussed their struggles with their illnesses. It was emotional, it was painful, but it was also exhilarating and enlightening."

Berman was a go-go, push-push type of guy, a fighter since childhood, when he was shuttled from foster home to foster home, having been given up for adoption when he was a year and a half old. But Friends in Deed taught him the value of slowing down.

"That group became my beacon for finding inner peace. I know this sounds really sixties, but that's what it was. Every Tuesday evening, I went to their meeting, meditated with them, and found myself feeling at first more relaxed, and later more refreshed and awake as a result. I could see the value of this in coping with the stress and trauma of a serious disease."

He would need his newfound relaxation techniques to cope with the next setback. In the fall of 1994, Lebow died. At the time of his original diagnosis in 1990, he had been given six months to live. He lived almost five more productive years. And of all the things he had created—a worldwide running organization of thirty-two thousand members, the great New York City Marathon, other events and races that were a part of the fabric of New York life—one of the things he was proudest of (he told Berman) was the Cancer Support Group for Athletes.

The program Lebow had encouraged Berman to start was now gaining momentum. They had outgrown the weekly meetings in the club and were now meeting twice a month at Mt. Sinai Medical Center, a major New York City cancer hospital, which validated the whole concept of what they were doing. Major New York hospitals were now expressing interest in starting similar programs; others began referring some of their own patients to Berman. Suddenly, Berman was on the front line of the war against cancer. To arm himself, he read, he attended lectures, he visited hospitals, and he talked with patients and physicians and other cancer-care experts and providers.

This led to another major change in his life. On July 23, 1995, after a long and bitter fight over disability benefits (those with cancer know all too well how unsympathetic some corporations and health insurers can be), Berman walked out of the media sales business for good.

"I knew at that point that my life was going to be about cancer. It sounds funny. You've heard of Bill Nye, the Science Guy? Well, in New York at least, I was becoming known as Jeff Berman, the Cancer Guy!"

But Jeff was a cancer guy with a plan, a program, and ideas that seemed to work. Soon, Berman was invited to set up support programs at Sloan-Kettering. His organization was awarded a $10,000 grant for innovation from the Zale Foundation. Then, in September 1996, Berman took a giant step. With the support of Mt. Sinai's Wellness Program, he developed and introduced a comprehensive, thirteen-week, three-part intervention program.

The Tuesday after Labor Day 1996, twenty-five women filed into a conference room at Mt. Sinai. All battling breast cancer, the women were of different ages and backgrounds and at different stages of dealing with their disease. Berman was there to meet them, along with his new staff: a nutritionist, an exercise physiologist, and a stress management specialist. A Mt. Sinai oncologist put it all in perspective for the cancer patients. The meeting began with Berman standing up.

"Congratulations for getting this far, for actually coming tonight. You've taken an important first step toward helping yourself. So welcome to our first meeting. Before we begin, I'd like to tell you a little story, about how I got here."

That night, the FORCE program was born.

CHAPTER TWO

THE FORCE PROGRAM: WHAT WE DO, HOW IT WORKS

In the 1960s, Dr. Kenneth Cooper, a senior flight surgeon and lieutenant colonel in the U.S. Air Force, began advocating a new kind of medicine, *preventive* medicine, based on vigorous exercise and proper diet.

Cooper even suggested that cardiac patients could benefit from this approach. At the time, the standard treatment for those who had suffered a heart attack was a soft chair, a comfy couch, and a quiet, sedentary life. Cooper, along with a few other like-minded physicians, preached something very different. He urged people to get up and get moving, to live vigorous, active lives, alter their diets by eating lots of fruits and vegetables, using skim instead of whole milk, and to limit consumption of red meats and egg yolks.

The naysayers, of whom there were many in the media and the medical community, called Cooper and folks who adopted similar philosophies "health nuts."

They were healthy, all right, but they were anything but nuts.

Cooper, of course, wasn't the first to advocate an active lifestyle. Doctors and other healers since Hippocrates himself have recommended exercise as part of the formula for a long and healthy life. But somehow, this message to patients became lost amid the dazzling technical achievements of modern medicine.

Today, Cooper's ideas are mainstream. Every major public health organization, including the U.S. Surgeon General's office, now recommends daily activity for all Americans. Now, people who have heart attacks are given an exercise prescription when they leave the cardiac care unit. They're told to exercise: moderately at first, and under the supervision of trained exercise physiologists. Cardiac patients—the "cardiac cripples" of thirty years ago—are now told to walk, to pedal stationary bikes, to move and use their bodies as part of their recovery treatment.

In treating everything from diabetes to depression, the medical community is beginning to recognize the value of physical activity, of strengthening the body through exercise *and* a proper diet. Physical activity has become a part of the treatment of almost every major disease except one.

Cancer.

The discussion of cancer treatments never seems to get past chemotherapy, radiation, and drugs. We believe there's another powerful source that can be tapped in to: the human body. Yes, even a body battling cancer can still get stronger, through exercise and diet and other lifestyle treatments. Although physical activity and a proper diet will not "cure" cancer or substitute for chemo or the medical interventions commonly prescribed by oncologists, these lifestyle approaches can play an important role in how fast and how well you recover from your disease or how well you coexist with it. As in the treatment of almost every other serious disease, an exercise regimen and good nutrition will help you in the treatment of cancer.

Is it a radical idea? We don't think so. As we've noted, a growing number of people in the cancer-fighting community believe this; growing numbers of recovering cancer patients already know it from their own experience. It makes perfect sense that the care of your body—what you do with it, what you put in it, how you treat it—is directly related to how effectively you can fight cancer.

THE FORCE PROGRAM:
WHO, WHAT, WHERE

Oncologists are big on presenting a strategy to cure your cancer. This typically involves a certain number of chemotherapy sessions and a certain number of doses of radiation and drugs. You've probably gotten something like this from your doctor: "50 rads or grays per day, M–F for six weeks." The FORCE program is designed to work in tandem with your doctor's. Developed in consultation with a group of professionals (exercise physiologists, nutritionists, stress management professionals, and oncologists), the FORCE program has been offered in New York City since September 1996. To date, more than three hundred people have completed the thirteen-week program. They're men and women who have ranged in age from twenty-four to eighty-five, from all backgrounds and professions, with all kinds of cancer and at varying stages of the disease. The vast majority of these FORCE graduates have adhered to the program—and though we can't say they've all been cured, we do know that those who have stuck with it have shown a marked improvement in their quality of life. Here's what a few graduates of the FORCE program told us about their experience:

"The FORCE program helped me to be more aware of what I can do with my life. Since graduating from the program three years ago, I have been cancer-free, and now I live each day with an appreciation of life and a hope that other people like me will join the FORCE program and learn and be motivated, much the way I was."

—*David Anderson, 64, Red Bank, New Jersey*
Prostate cancer survivor, FORCE graduate '98

"The average person with cancer usually doesn't know what to do. The FORCE program showed us. We studied nutrition; we were directly exposed to and involved with the various aspects of the program. Instead of a one-sentence reference telling us that 'You should pay attention to your nutrition' and so forth, Jeff and his colleagues gave us everything we needed to know. It was great. I would highly recommend it."

—*Arthur Pogran, 88, New York City*
Prostate cancer survivor, FORCE graduate '98

"The FORCE program sounds like just what the doctor ordered. The reality is, however, that beyond diagnosis, surgery, chemotherapy, and radiation, most doctors really don't have much advice to give. The FORCE program fills a critical need in showing you the importance of good nutrition, developing a specialized exercise plan, and teaching you ways of coping with stress. The amazing thing is that many people complete this program while they are still on chemo, learning the tools and gaining the hope for a new, cancer-free life."

—*Barbara Morgan, 49, New York City*
Breast cancer survivor, FORCE graduate, '99

The media have also taken notice of the FORCE program. We were honored to be listed as an "innovative exercise program" in the January 2001 issue of Dr. Andrew Weil's *Self-Healing* newsletter. The program and founder Jeff Berman have also been featured in the *New York Times*, the *Washington Post*, the *Los Angeles Times*, *New York Newsday*, and the *Miami Herald*, as well as on local television news programs.

FORCE is the only program of its type in the country that is not conducted exclusively in a hospital or health club setting. Our patients spend a few hours a week with us, then do the rest at home, on their own, which is exactly what you can do.

FORCE covers three basic areas:

- *Exercise:* An individualized program of aerobic and weight-bearing exercise that varies depending on the patient's age and condition and the nature of the patient's disease. Don't worry: We're not telling you that you have to bench-press your body weight or run a marathon. We start gradually, we start slowly, but in every case we've seen, people start to feel better when they follow the program. And so will you.
- *Stress Management:* Reducing stress will help anyone become less anxious and more willing to make positive changes in habits and lifestyle. So stress reduction is particularly important for people with cancer. Our four-week stress management recommendations will help you manage the unique pressures and emotional issues that arise with cancer. We've been there; we understand; and we can teach some techniques that can help you feel better and a little more together.
- *Nutrition:* FORCE patients get four weeks of nutritional counseling, once a week for an hour. The goal is to help patients learn how to maintain proper caloric intake during treatment, to better develop nutritional habits known to reduce the risks of certain types of cancer and prevent recurrence. Patients are also taught how to shop and read labels and how to prepare healthier foods.

We're going to go into more detail about each of these areas in the following chapters, and we will show you how to tailor a program that's right for you. But first, let's talk about what's going on upstairs.

We're not going to kid you: Following this prescription takes discipline, hard work, and determination. That's why the first step in the FORCE program is getting yourself into the right frame of mind.

STEP ONE: GET YOUR HEAD ON STRAIGHT

"You've got cancer."

These are the words everyone dreads.

We know how it feels to hear those words: you're shocked, you're devastated, you feel like the foundations of your life have just given way beneath you, and you're plummeting fast.

You're expected to have those kinds of feelings. Cancer is, after all, a serious disease. But don't wallow in those negative emotions; don't let them rule your life. Remember: There are still things—many things, important things—that are within your control. Things you can do to help your situation. That's what the FORCE program is all about. But before we get to working with your muscles, we've got to deal with your mind.

Here are our FORCE principles for getting yourself into the right frame of mind to fight your cancer. Please learn them and live by them. You'll find that using them will dramatically improve your ability to deal with your disease, and your success in making the lifestyle changes we outline in this book will be greatly enhanced.

DRY THOSE TEARS . . . AND FIRE UP YOUR ENGINES

You've wept, you've pounded the desk with your fists, you've asked God "Why me?" We don't mean to minimize those feelings. They're real and genuine and it's important that you have them and recognize them. As we just said, they are the first and natural reaction for anyone who has had the disease. But enough's enough. It's time to move on.

Now you have to take what we call our Patton approach. That's the disciplinarian General George S. Patton of World War II fame. Take out a (figurative) glove and slap yourself across the face three times. Okay? You needed that, didn't you? Right. Now remind yourself that there are things you can do and that there is work to be done. Productive, positive work that you yourself must do. Let's get to it.

TELL YOURSELF "I CAN"

Norman Vincent Peale popularized the truth about the power of positive thinking. You can use this power in your own life and as part of your own treatment.

Maybe right now the thought of trying to modify your diet or begin a walking program sounds tough. And it may be tough. But don't give us this "I can't" stuff. We have seen people with advanced, inoperable cancers, the elderly, the weak, the never-did-any-exercise-before crowd—people in worse condition than yours—take and meet the FORCE challenge.

Most of them have survived—and you can, too. But you've got to remind yourself that you're capable of it. You can get better. You can feel better. Tell yourself, right now, "I can."

ASK QUESTIONS, EXPECT ANSWERS

We hope that most or all of your questions about the role of movement and lifestyle in cancer treatment will be answered in this book. But we also know that every case is individual, and that there are aspects about your situation that are different from the next person's. The one individual who can best answer your questions about your treatment and your situation is your oncologist. When you speak, is your oncologist listening? If not, get his or her attention. Today's physicians—the good ones, at least—expect questions, and should be willing to answer yours. So ask already. You're not sure when to take the medicine? Ask. You're not sure about the side effects of your chemo? Ask. And if the information is still not forthcoming or sufficient, refer to the next steps.

DO YOUR HOMEWORK

If you're reading a book like this, chances are you're the type of person who's hungry for information about your disease and how to fight it. One of the things Lance Armstrong said that he felt was key in his successful battle against testicular cancer was simply finding out more about it. He recommends that people with cancer gather information, visit the library, get on the Internet. You want to learn about the latest medicines, the latest advances, the drugs that are being prescribed.

We echo and emphasize that advice. In our appendix, we list some good Web sites and resources for cancer patients. Explore them. They may provide you with additional information that can help you better deal with your disease.

USE THE OPPORTUNITY CANCER HAS GIVEN YOU

We hear you scoffing. "*Opportunity?* This disease has turned my life upside down, terrified me, put me through the indignities of invasive medical treatments—and you think it's something positive?"

Well, yeah. Cancer gives you the opportunity to get your life in shape, to reevaluate where you are putting precious energy that you need for yourself and your recovery. Do you have some high-maintenance friends who are using up too much of your energy right now? Maybe it's time to ice those friendships, or redefine them. Were you pondering a job change, thinking about a move, or even looking for an excuse to take guitar lessons or volunteer at the local museum? Cancer creates a unique opportunity for you to make these changes (some of which may have been long overdue!) and to boost your mood by doing things that make you feel good.

We're not suggesting you do these things because "time is short." In fact, cancer mortality rates have dropped over the past five years. Rather, we say this because we know that cancer has a wonderful way of concentrating the mind, of sifting out what's important and what's not, of setting and resetting priorities. Do it—you'll be happier, which, in turn, will help you better fight your disease.

DON'T GET OVERPROTECTED

At the request of a friend, Jeff Berman called a man who was ill with cancer to tell him about the FORCE program. His wife answered the phone.

"What's this about?" she asked, reluctant to put her husband on the phone.

"The FORCE program," said Berman.

"What's that?" she asked suspiciously.

"It's a program that involves, among other things, exercise for cancer patients," he explained.

"Oh," she said. "He's too sick for that." Click.

That woman's instinct was one we can all understand. She wanted to protect her husband, just as your family and friends are probably feeling protective about you right now. That's wonderful and that's why we love them. But it's counterproductive if they begin to decide, as this woman obviously did, what *you* can and can't do. Only you know that. As our good friend Dr. Steve Jonas, professor of preventive medicine at the State University of New York/Stony Brook Medical School, likes to say, "Explore your limits, know your limitations."

Let's explore.

LIGHTEN UP

"Laughter is the best medicine," claimed Norman Cousins. He was right. Although we don't know of any psychological study on this, we would bet (and our anecdotal experience as cancer patient and caregiver supports this) that the cancer patients who do best tend to be those who can laugh. At themselves. At us. At the world. These are the survivors who recover and enjoy their lives.

When Jeff was first diagnosed in 1990, some of his well-meaning friends actually suggested he see the film *Dying Young.* Instead, he went out and rented Mel Brooks's *The Producers* and *Monty Python and the Holy Grail.* You should rent or read whatever appeals to your sense of humor, whether that's Pink Panther movies or *Dumb and Dumber.* (Cousins himself watched the Marx Brothers.)

TAKE RESPONSIBILITY FOR YOUR HEALTH

Your doctor, your spouse, your family, and your friends can do only so much. The rest is up to you. Because you're reading this book, chances are you're motivated enough to want to take at least part of your treatment into your own hands. That's good, because nobody knows you better than you.

The good news is that there are things you can do—outside of the hospital or the treatment center—to help yourself. The FORCE program is one of those things that will strengthen your mind, body, and spirit. So let's get started on it.

First, pat yourself on the back. You've awakened yourself to the need for action with the glove in the face. Now, you should give yourself some credit, because you've already done something positive. You've taken action by reading this book.

By patting yourself on the back you're also now in touch with the one person who must ultimately take the responsibility for getting you healthy again. Others can help, but in the end, it's up to you to take charge of your battle against this disease.

Yes, you've got cancer. Now, it's time to start fighting back.

STEP TWO: EXERCISE AND PHYSICAL ACTIVITY

Our exercise physiologist, John Buzzerio, hates the word "exercise." He's not alone. Epidemiologist Steve Blair, the senior scientist on the historic Surgeon

General's *Report on Exercise and Physical Activity* in 1996, also makes the distinction. Here's how he defines it:

- *Exercise* is planned, repetitive activity with a goal toward building fitness and sports performance.
- *Physical activity* is energy expenditure by human movement through routine daily activity.

Are you ready to exercise? Maybe, maybe not. Maybe the thought of exercise frightens you. Maybe you think you can't do anything really strenuous right now. Or maybe you're already involved in some form of physical activity. Either way, you should understand that not everyone in the FORCE program starts out by doing "exercise." Many of them begin by engaging in "physical activity," simply putting one foot in front of the other. Case in point:

A cousin of Buzzerio's had cancer. While she was undergoing chemo, she came to him and the FORCE program for help. John wanted to see what she could do and found out that the answer was "not much."

"Her exercise program was to do two laps around her dining room table," he said. "That was it. And she couldn't make it the first time. I held her by her wrist and helped her through one and a half laps. Then she had to stop."

That was her "baseline": one lap around the dining room. And yet, from that humble beginning, Buzzerio's cousin, whose disease was serious, can now walk several blocks, unassisted. She started slow, very slow, but she improved. And she feels better. So will you.

(By the way, John's cousin is now disease-free. Her participation in the FORCE program didn't cure her, but it sure helped her recovery.)

Your exercise—make that "physical activity"—may be walking. Or it may involve just picking up the groceries unassisted, or climbing the stairs, or mowing your lawn. On the other hand, it could involve fun stuff like dancing, skating, and hiking, as well as more vigorous activities, such as running, cycling, and weight training.

We'll help you get there. In the FORCE program, we have a fourteen-week exercise program involving different types of activities. When people think of exercise, they think of walking, running, bicycling. That's only one kind of exercise—called aerobics—and it helps strengthen your heart and cardiovascular and immune systems. However, we also emphasize another form of exercise in the FORCE program: strengthening. No, we're not going to order you to the gym and demand that you start churning out reps on a Hammer strength machine. We *are* going to remind you, however, that strengthening your muscles is vital for your continued quality of life. It's important that you are strong enough to carry your groceries, for instance, stand steadily in the shower, and get yourself out of a tub. The movements you need to do for this important kind of strength training are basic, particularly in the beginning stages of the program, and can be done at home, on your own, and without a lot of fancy equipment. And it can work.

Remember: One of the best studies on exercise and cancer showed that cancer patients on a ten-week exercise program increased their strength by an average of 43 percent and doubled the amount of time they spent on aerobic exercise. Doubled! These are people with cancer, like you.

That means you can do it, too. You *can* increase your strength; you *can* get in better shape. You can do it even with your disease and even if you're not in shape now. We want you to feel this wonderful news in your body and mind: You can still get strong. Your body has not totally betrayed you. Take that, cancer!

STEP THREE: STRESS MANAGEMENT

Stress is often defined as our body's response to change. Stress is not inherently bad. If we didn't have a "stress mechanism"—the so-called fight-or-flight response—most of our ancestors would have ended up as the main entree for hungry saber-toothed tigers instead of running away from them or, eventually, figuring out how to stop them.

There is good stress and there is bad stress. Chances are, if you've been diagnosed with cancer, most of your stress lately has been bad. But we can tell you some good ways to fight that bad stress. Our FORCE patients learn some very basic but very effective stress management techniques over their four weeks with our stress management expert, Bette Jean Rosenhagen. This book will teach you these same mind-body techniques: basic deep-breathing exercises and visualization and relaxation techniques. You can learn these on your own, at your own pace.

These techniques help you change your response to stress. By learning something called "mindfulness-based" meditation, you will be able to stay in the moment and become more aware of yourself, your options, and your strengths. It's a way to find moments of clarity during daily stresses or challenges. And boy, can that be valuable.

We're not saying we can teach you how to yawn in the face of the saber-toothed tigers and other threats that prowl our modern jungles. Indeed, we don't want you to be indifferent to all stresses or to ignore them. There are times when you may need to get angry and fight instead of flee, such as when dealing with inconsiderate friends, an insensitive boss, or insurance agencies. At such times, feeling "stressed" can be a positive motivator. Generally, you'll find that your ability to manage the demands of your job, your family, and your disease—not to mention your ability to stick with other aspects of the FORCE program, such as modifying your diet or sticking with an exercise regimen—will be enhanced once you learn some mind-body techniques. They will help you deal more effectively with the life challenges you're experiencing.

Stress management is simply learning how to react to circumstances you can't change. It is also learning to see how to change things that you can. For example, you can learn to change how you react to having cancer (Remember: "I *can* get better!"). Learning not to get yourself twisted into a pretzel over things you can't control, such as the fact that you have cancer, is important. Accepting that you have it and accepting that you can help yourself get rid of it will give you the peace and clarity of mind you need to do the things you can do to fight it.

A recent study at Ohio State University found that women who participated in a stress management program similar to the FORCE program showed lower levels of stress hormone and higher levels of an antibody that fights breast tumors than patients who did not learn how to reduce their stress. The women who learned and practiced the stress management techniques not only felt better, they *were* better—physically and emotionally. "We're finding that stress and distress can be significantly reduced in breast cancer patients and that these effects are linked to lowering of a stress hormone, a stronger immune response, and a better quality of life," said Dr. Barbara Andersen, a professor at Ohio State and the leader of the study.

STEP FOUR: LET'S EAT (BETTER)

It seems that you can't open a magazine, turn on your TV, or have a conversation without hearing about the latest miracle diet cures, the hottest fad sports performance diet, the supplement that allows someone to hit seventy home runs.

At the FORCE program, we try to sidestep all that. We're not interested in selling any particular nutritional supplements or foods (there is not, and will never be, a "FORCE Bar"). We're not interested in getting in the middle of the "carbs are good, carbs are the enemy" debate that you can find in any gym. We are interested in what the scientific research shows about cancer and nutrition. Heather Salomon, a registered dietitian and bionutritionist, works with our FORCE patients over a four-week period, sharing her extensive and practical knowledge of nutrition and cancer. Heather has developed diets, menus, and guidelines for patients with various types of cancer. She also has a basic nutritional philosophy for all cancer patients, one that emphasizes common sense. In our groups—and for you, our readers—we'll focus on these key aspects of nutrition and cancer. Here are a few of the tips we'll provide and the issues we'll clarify:

- *Fruits, vegetables, and fiber:* As the USDA food pyramid depicts, these are the foundation of a good diet. But for cancer patients, there is a special added significance to these foods: they contain phytochemicals, naturally occurring, disease-fighting chemicals in plant-based foods. Phytochemicals have been shown to be important cancer fighters on the cellular level.
- *Fats:* Most epidemiological studies have shown that a low-fat diet is better for prevention of cancer. We'll explain how low is low, and what types of fats you should avoid.
- *Soy:* Deserving of its own focus for many reasons, but especially because of its powerful phytoestrogens, which are cancer fighters.
- *Supplements and herbal remedies:* Can they help? In some cases, perhaps. But there's a lot of hype and misinformation out there about these products. Our other FORCE program nutritionist, Douglas Kalman, MS, RD, looks at the most popular and shows you which ones are beneficial.

Finally, and perhaps most important, you need to know how to use all this nutritional information. After we've explained which kinds of food you should be eating and what kind of diet you should be following, we give you the same hints and tips that our patients in the weekly FORCE nutrition sessions get. In fact, in our face-to-face weekly meetings, we take our patients on a grocery store field trip. We'll do something similar for you in our nutrition chapter in a "virtual" shopping trip. We'll walk you down the aisles of a typical supermarket and tell you where to stop and what to avoid. You can bring this book along when you go shopping so that you can make sure you're getting the foods we recommend in the FORCE program, the foods that can help your body fight cancer.

CHAPTER THREE

GETTING STARTED

Your first assignment in the FORCE program: Get your doctor's permission.

Perhaps that's easier said than done. Perhaps you find intimidating the idea of marching into your oncologist's office and telling him or her that you're going to start following a program outside of the treatments he or she has already recommended. So first, let's talk about the relationship of the cancer patient and the physician. It's a complex and sometimes challenging relationship, but an essential one. (And remember, the authors of this book represent both sides of this relationship: Jeff Berman is a patient and Dr. Fran Fleegler is an oncologist.)

Let's start with the day that you received the dreaded news. Getting a diagnosis of cancer is like being on a ship that has inadvertently sailed into a storm, with you at the helm. Not necessarily "the Perfect Storm," one from which there is little chance of escape, but a stiff nor'easter that's going to challenge your skills and your resolve.

As a person with cancer, you must make it your job to take the wheel, to help steer the strategy for treatment and recovery. Just as a sailor might freeze at the first sight of the impending storm, many patients feel frozen in a state of inaction by the negative emotions and anxiety surrounding their diagnosis. Complicating matters, a person with cancer is frequently surrounded by a "crew" of advisors, all with good intent, who may attempt to point you in "the right direction." To top it all off, you're likely to be swamped by information about cancer and related issues.

In an ideal world, your relationship with your oncologist would be open and would allow you the time and space to be involved in all aspects of mapping out your treatment. In an ideal world, your doctor would want to read about the FORCE program and volunteer to serve as your personal coach and cheerleader as you begin. Your doctor would share inspirational anecdotes of patients already using the FORCE program and offer to connect you with them. "How can we integrate the FORCE program into our treatment plan?" the doctor would ask.

Well, it should be no surprise to you that most doctors may not initially share your enthusiasm for a new fitness program. The doctor is often too concerned about the white blood cell count, your body surface area, or some other term or procedure or value that will often end up sounding like medical gobbledygook.

What you need to do, first and foremost, is develop a strategy for communicating with your doctor, one that allows you to form a true therapeutic and healing partnership as you go into cancer therapy. This partnership must be based on openness, honesty, and trust. And the doctor should be your cocaptain on the cancer treatment team.

Physicians who are board-certified cancer specialists are highly qualified, rigorously trained professionals who have at least five years of training beyond medical school. Oncology specialists also continue to educate themselves by reading the latest medical studies and attending meetings and symposia. From a purely objective standpoint, doctors who care for patients with cancer are dedicated to the mission of healing and will be able to outline a treatment plan individually tailored to your needs. Your doctor will know how to effectively administer chemotherapy as well as blood products and other supportive medications.

When it comes to a therapeutic healing relationship with your doctor, however, diplomas, certifications, and objective competency are not the only important factors. Undertaking cancer treatment, no matter where it leads, requires insight, sensitivity, trust, thoughtfulness, patience, and compassion. Wouldn't it be wonderful if we could assume that every oncology specialist was endowed with these humanistic qualities? But the truth is, more times than not, you will need to capture your doctor's attention to gain his or her support, and perhaps even enthusiasm, for the FORCE program.

Oncologists actually have a great interest in learning about complementary approaches in cancer care. They are deluged with information from the Internet, magazine articles, and television news blurbs. The doctor's problem, as is yours, is to sift through all the weird, bizarre, and sometimes potentially harmful material to find helpful cancer-fighting tips.

There is ample evidence that both patients and physicians feel greater satisfaction with the treatment experience when their communication is open and relaxed. Doctors *want* to be perceived as compassionate and caring listeners. However, doctors are notorious for interrupting your spoken thoughts, avoiding eye contact, or even standing with their hand on the doorknob as you try to ask a question (talk about communicating with body language!). A study that appeared in a leading oncology journal in 1999 was entitled "Can 40 Seconds of Compassion Reduce Patient Anxiety?" The answer was a resounding yes! But forty seconds in the heat of a busy day may seem like a precious commodity to your doctor. Here's how to make sure you command the attention you deserve when you discuss the FORCE program with him or her:

- Have an agenda for your doctor-patient meeting. Plan in advance. Bring a list.
- Make both physical contact and eye contact. Shake her hand. Look him in the eye.
- Tell your doctor about the FORCE program. Tell him or her that this is your personal Race for the Cure, not to mention a good way to get into some healthy habits.
- Inform your cancer care specialist that you want to take some responsibility for remaining fit and healthy while undergoing treatment.
- Enlist your doctor's support. Assure him or her that you will review highlights as the program proceeds, and that the doctor will remain the captain of your whole program. That will make for smoother sailing for everyone!

YOUR PART OF THE BARGAIN

Cancer or no cancer, change does not come easily to us humans. Ask the estimated six out of ten people who try to start an exercise program every year and fail. Ask the one out of four Americans who is totally sedentary, doing absolutely nothing, despite the consensus that exercise and a healthy diet are important to health. Most of these folks don't even have cancer or any serious disease, and they're still on the couch. No, siree, it's not easy. But we've got some ideas on how to make it easier: suggestions that will motivate you further and that can help you start and stick with the regimen of exercise and diet and stress management that make up the FORCE program.

It's all about *change.* James Prochaska, Ph.D., is an expert in change. A psychologist and author, Prochaska heads up the Health Promotion Partnership at the University of Rhode Island and has been instrumental in developing a model of change that has been used successfully by thousands of people. *Health* magazine reported on Prochaska's model in its January 2000 issue, and recommended that people follow it, particularly those people looking to make good on their New Year's fitness resolutions. Well, the way we see it, you're looking to make a New *Life* resolution. A New Life after cancer. So you'd be wise to understand it, too.

STAGE 1: PRECONTEMPLATION

At this stage, you're unconvinced you need to change. Chances are *you* are past this stage if you're reading this now.

STAGE 2: CONTEMPLATION

Health magazine notes that this is the stage where a lot of people who want to embark on a fitness program find themselves stuck. Maybe you know there are things you should do, but you're having trouble figuring out how to do them, how to find the time, how to put your car into drive. Some people get stuck here for a while. Contemplation becomes procrastination, and eventually the whole idea of change is abandoned.

The rest go on to the next stage.

STAGE 3: PREPARATION

This is where you make a plan. And this is where we can help. We've got a plan for you to follow—the FORCE plan—which is detailed step-by-step in this book. We'll give you all the general principles of the program, plus variations you can use depending on your type and stage of cancer.

STAGE 4: ACTION

You could also call this the Nike step, after the famous Nike ad slogan "Just Do It." Prochaska would argue that just doing it isn't enough for some people, if they haven't already gone through the other stages. But now, with a purpose and a plan, you should be ready to take action.

STAGE 5: MAINTENANCE

This is where you form the habit. This is where you go from being somebody new at exercise to being a regular exerciser. This is where it becomes like brushing your teeth: something you do naturally, even joyfully.

STAGE 6: TERMINATION

You've put the past behind you. You've changed, my friend. Welcome to the next stage of your life.

LET'S GET GOING!

Most of the people we meet coming into the FORCE program are somewhere between Stages 2 and 3. They're contemplating making the changes we recommend, but they need a road map, and they need someone sitting beside them, like their Driver Ed instructor back in high school, to encourage, guide, and support them.

That's where we come in. We have the plan: an exercise, diet, and stress management plan you can follow and modify to your particular needs. And we'll be there, right here, every step of the way. (And if the printed page is too impersonal, you can contact us in person. We've included information on how to do that in the Resources section of this book.) The FORCE program can help you immediately, even if you are still going through treatment. We can help lessen your anxiety with some proven stress-reduction techniques, we can help you begin to make some of the necessary dietary modifications, and yes, we can even get you started on exercise. And, unless your physician has specifically forbidden it, we don't want to hear "I can't do it now. I have to wait." Almost everyone reading this book should be able to do something. And if there's one thing we know about exercise and physical activity, it is that doing *something* is better—much, much better—than doing nothing.

Don't let yourself think that you can't do anything because of your disease. Case in point: Our friend and FORCE graduate Richard Shaffer was fifty-seven when he was hospitalized for metastasized melanoma. One evening, his sister Barbara paid him a late visit, around 10 P.M. She arrived in her brother's room to find an empty bed. Then, she heard grunting and groaning. Alarmed, she raced to the other side of the bed to find Dick doing push-ups. "What are you doing?" she asked. "I can't remember a day when I didn't stretch and do my push-ups and sit-ups. Why should today be any different?"

No surprise that, with that kind of discipline, Dick is doing great today, ten years later. Now, we're not saying you've got to climb out of your bed and start doing deep knee bends. But we are saying that if you want to take control over your disease, you have to take action, even small actions, to start. Following are some tips to help get you moving.

STARTING AND STICKING
WITH THE FORCE PROGRAM

MAKE A CONTRACT WITH YOURSELF

When you enter the FORCE program, which involves thirteen weekly meetings, you fill out a binding, ironclad, no-escape contract. This contract is not with us, not with our attorneys, not with your physician or health professional. Your contract is with *you*. Patients think they have to fill it out and hand it to Jeff Berman. He hands it right back and tells them they've made this deal with themselves. If they break the contract, they're breaking their own trust.

The language of this contract can be as simple and cogent as telling yourself, "I promise to follow this program for at least thirteen weeks." Or it can be a little more involved; you can specify each aspect of the program and commit yourself to it. Type it up, print it out, sign it, and then stick it up on your bulletin board or your refrigerator. You'll be amazed at the power of a written agreement—especially one with yourself.

I pledge that I will exercise regularly, gradually building up to three to four times a week, and that I will follow the dietary guidelines and practice the stress management techniques of the FORCE program. I resolve that I will perform my exercise safely and correctly, but consistently. I will not let social or work activities interfere with my training schedule, and if obligations arise that must be met, I promise that I will find time at another point of the day to do my exercise or that I will make up the workout the next day. I furthermore pledge that I will maintain the schedule outlined in this book for thirteen to sixteen weeks (depending on how quickly I progress through the phases of the exercise program).

At the end of that time, I will renegotiate these terms.

Your signature

START SMALL AND FOCUS ON CONSISTENCY

Some folks holler "Charge!" and rush into an exercise program like Pickett's troops charging the Union lines at Gettysburg. And you know what happened to those guys. (Memo to those who slept through history class: Pickett's Confederates were repulsed; they lost the battle and the Civil War.)

Very often, new exercisers will work hard, very hard at the beginning, logging hours in the gym, doing this, doing that, and then . . . flash! They fizzle and burn out like a Roman candle. Much better to take small steps. As personal trainers like to tell their out-of-shape clients, "It took you thirty years to get out of shape, so it's going to take you more than three weeks to get back into shape."

That's true, especially when you might be coming back not only from a sedentary lifestyle, but from cancer and the toxicity of the treatment as well.

Your best bet? Start gradually. Make consistency your goal. As we'll discuss in our chapter on exercise, you can begin to feel the benefits of exercise with a relatively small amount of work. In fact, we've had FORCE patients who've started by walking for as little as five minutes. That's all you need to get going.

WRITE IT DOWN

Keeping a training log is one of the simplest and most effective ways to chart your progress and stay motivated. As with your contract, it doesn't have to be complex. Simply note the date, the workout—what you did, how hard, and for how long—and how you felt. You might also want to keep a daily diary of the foods you're eating (more about that in our chapter on nutrition). You'll find that as the days go on, you'll be walking or cycling for a longer amount of time, and you'll feel and see yourself getting stronger—in black and white. A training log provides irrefutable proof of progress to the most important person in the FORCE program: you. Even more important, it serves as a reminder that on this front of your war against cancer, *you* are the one in control.

SET A TIME FOR EXERCISE, AND DON'T BE LATE!

It's been shown that people are more likely to stick with a program if they do it on a set day and time, as opposed to "squeezing it in" whenever they can. Of course, time is a big issue for all of us. Bottom line: You can make the time. We don't care how busy you are, if it's important enough to you, you can make the time. And what's more important than your health?

Some people write their exercise time down in their appointment book. "Wednesday, 7 A.M.: Ride exercise bike for 30 minutes." It's a good technique, because it underscores your workout's importance. You wouldn't blow off a meet-

ing scheduled with an important client, right? Well, think of your exercise appointment the same way.

SHARE THE LOAD

Training partners make exercise more sociable, more pleasant, more bearable,
particularly on those inevitable days when you just don't feel like getting out of
bed. They also make us hold up our end of the bargain. You can find a training
partner almost anywhere: at work, in your neighborhood, in a chat room, by
posting a notice at your local health club. Some folks even find their training
partners in their own home (a spouse, a parent, a child).

Don't worry if your training partner has cancer or not. Far more important
is that your training partner is someone who is at about your level of fitness,
someone who is as committed as you are, and someone whose company you
enjoy.

FIND SOMETHING YOU LIKE

Sounds obvious, right? Maybe not. An out-of-shape friend of one of the coauthors started an exercise program a few years ago. This fellow, a big guy, decided to run, which was probably not the best choice of exercise for him. But he
ran and ran on the treadmill at his health club. "How's your running coming?"
we asked after a few weeks. "Great," he panted. "I hate it." Huh? "Well, I know this
isn't supposed to be fun, right?" Wrong. Sure, exercise by definition involves effort, but you shouldn't be dreading it. Loathe it for long, and you won't end up
doing it for long. Remember: There's something out there for you. Even if it's
something as basic as walking. And you can create an environment—with the
company of other people or by watching TV or listening to music while you
exercise—that can make any activity more pleasurable.

P.S. Our friend took up cycling, which was much better suited to his body type. He enjoys his bike rides. And maybe because of that, he's stuck with it years later.

GET YOUR FAMILY INTO—OR OUT OF—THE PROCESS

When Berman was diagnosed in 1990, his mom offered this advice: "Don't lift anything heavy. Don't run around. Take it easy." Mama Berman just wanted to protect her son, a reaction typical of many family members. To some extent, this impulse to look out for you is part of a loving relationship. But to the extent that this protectiveness keeps you from taking action and making these important changes, they are counterproductive. You'll have to analyze people's reactions on a case-by-case basis. Although we strongly recommend that you try to get your family involved in helping you with the FORCE program, we understand that in reality that might not happen, simply because of the complex psychological issues that cancer raises within families. So, if your spouse/parents/kids/family are behind your effort to make changes, to start exercising and modifying your diet, great. Welcome aboard. If they're ambivalent or if they even begin to serve as a barrier, then you're just going to have to work around them for the time being.

Your efforts at making major lifestyle changes may prompt different reactions within your own family. Some members may be in favor of your going out for your long walk on a chilly day; others may be barring the door to keep you inside, in a well-intentioned but misguided attempt to protect you. We recommend that you listen to the voices of encouragement and tune out the voices of discouragement. Ultimately, you have to do what's best for you. And getting active, getting stronger, adapting a more healthful diet: *This* is what's best for you. Indeed, for all of us.

CHAPTER FOUR

STRESS MANAGEMENT

S tress. We see it in the face of all the patients who join the FORCE program. They all have the stress of dealing with their disease, their treatment, their lives.

You can expect to feel stress when you have cancer. The diagnosis, the treatment, the emotional roller coaster, the whole rigmarole of dealing with cancer is stressful. But many patients believe that stress somehow *caused* their cancer.

Is it true? No, stress itself does not cause cancer.

That's not to say that accumulated, negative stress over a long period of time—combined with other unhealthy behaviors, such as smoking, lack of exercise, and poor diet—can't have negative health consequences. There is some evidence that people who are "stressed out" have a suppressed immune system, which can lead to a greater susceptibility to infections and even to some neurological diseases. The stresses of job and family keep many people from maintaining their health by keeping doctor's appointments and getting regular exercise and eating properly. Stress drives some to do things they shouldn't, such as smoke or drink alcohol to excess. Although some of these behaviors can contribute to certain forms of cancer—the link between smoking and lung cancer, for example, is well established—no expert has demonstrated a direct link between stress and cancer.

It's human nature to find something or someone to blame when things go wrong. So, when faced with a diagnosis of cancer, we immediately "go negative." We ask ourselves, "What did I do wrong?" High stress levels qualify as a convenient culprit. The real suspects in most cancer cases—genes or chromosomes—make for poor villains: they're too abstract, too tiny. Although we can't see stress, we can sure feel its effects: our stomach rumbles, our head aches, our teeth grind, and our neck and shoulders feel as tight as if they're being pinched by a giant pair of calipers. So, we assume, if stress can do all that to our bodies, it might give us cancer, too.

But it doesn't. Unlike cancer, all stress is not necessarily bad. Also, not everyone has cancer, but just about everyone deals with stress. As our FORCE stress management consultant Bette Jean Rosenhagen points out to our patients, "If stress causes cancer, the entire country would have cancer." Fortunately, that's not the case.

A SHORT HISTORY OF STRESS

It all started about forty thousand years ago. A Cro-Magnon man is standing outside his cave, minding his own business. Mrs. Cro-Magnon (people had hyphenated last names even then) calls out in prehistoric grunts, "Frank, watch out for that rock!" Mr. Cro-Magnon looks up, sees the rock tumbling down the hillside right for him. His body must become galvanized to act—to move out of the way—or he's prehistoric roadkill. So what happens? His pulse rate quickens, his mouth gets dry, his muscles tense up, adrenaline floods through his system. A quick evasive move, and his life is spared. Chalk up one for stress. Faced with certain death, or an injury rendering our friend unable to hunt, stress elicits a response to survive. This is an example of "good" stress, life-saving stress, the fight-or-flight response to stress articulated.

Now, what if there had been no stress? What if Mr. Cro-Magnon and all his brethren had been so mellow, calm, and relaxed that when they saw the rock, or the charging saber-toothed tiger, they just stood there and grunted in Cro-Magnonese, "Whatever"? Well, if that were the case, you wouldn't be reading this now, and we'd probably be walking around on all fours and paying homage to a flag with a saber-toothed tiger on it.

You see the point. There's positive stress and negative stress. Again, as Bette Jean likes to point out to our stressed-out FORCE patients, "If it wasn't for stress, you wouldn't get up in the morning. You wouldn't strive to achieve on your job, or to be a better parent." She's right. No stress, no pyramids, no Shakespeare plays, no Declaration of Independence, no Empire State Building, no nothing. So instead of blaming stress for your cancer, instead of seeing stress as the enemy, instead of the futile attempt to live a "stress-free" life, why don't you look at it the other way? Maybe the fight-or-flight response can help you do just that: fight back. Maybe stress can actually help you "beat" cancer. Faced with a diagnosis of cancer—today's version of the rock tumbling toward you—maybe you should "go Cro" (Magnon) and let this most basic human instinct work for you, instead of against you. Remember that prehistoric humans used their flight instinct (or stress response) and intelligence to survive and go on to build Civilization As We Know It. They forged ahead. We recommend doing the same. Strike out on a forward pathway: Work on getting better and feeling better. Set your mind on that one goal, and stop stressing out about whether stress caused your cancer. Instead, learn how to harness the good power of stress and work on reducing its bad effects. We can show you some simple ways to do just that.

STRESS MANAGEMENT IN THE FORCE PROGRAM

The first thing we work on in the FORCE program is stress reduction. Why? Because we believe that if you're too stressed when you start the program, you're likely to try to do too much too fast. Remember the tortoise and the hare? We'd rather that you make the lifestyle changes like the tortoise—in a controlled, slow, and deliberate way—and not emulate the hare, who goes too fast and burns out before getting to the finish line.

Even while balancing the rigors of treatment, people who follow our four-week stress-reduction course here in the FORCE program—people who take the "tortoise" approach to changing their diet and exercise habits—find it easier to make these permanent and long-lasting changes. The folks who dive right into it, who radically alter their diet and try to do monster workouts night after night, usually end up getting discouraged and frustrated. That harelike approach doesn't work, we suspect, because these folks are so pressured, so stressed that they demand too much too soon from their bodies and themselves.

The FORCE program tries to get folks balanced, centered. The techniques we teach in our four stress management sessions are simple. You can do them anywhere. They will help you manage stress and use it to your advantage. Think of the techniques as a sort of "mental judo," a way of managing stress the same way that masters of this ancient Japanese fighting art mastered their opponents. Judo (or jujitsu) does not require great physical strength; it involves utilizing your opponent's energy and movements to your advantage. Think of stress as an opponent that you don't need to defeat, but whose energy you want to utilize for your own benefit. Unlike judo, you don't have to learn any flips, holds, or falls. All you have to do to start is take a deep breath.

FORCE STRESS REDUCTION PROGRAM

STEP 1: BREATHE DEEPLY

Recently, we saw the best-selling author and physician Andrew Weil talk about how he became involved in holistic medicine. He recalled the time he asked one of his mentors, an osteopath, about the secret of good health. "He responded by taking a deep breath," recalled Weil. That was the "secret": A key to improved health is conscious breathing.

This ridiculously simple-sounding idea resonates through many cultures. In their book *The Essentials of Yoga,* Dinabandhu Sarley and Ila Sarley show how the importance of breath—beyond its primary and obvious importance in delivering oxygen to the body—is reflected in our language. Ennobling words such as "aspire" and "inspire" are derived from a Latin word, *spiritus:* "the breath of a God." In yoga, the concept of *prana,* the essential life force, is closely linked with breathing. The simple act of breathing links us with the flow and rhythm of life itself. We don't get too philosophical about this in the FORCE program, but we do agree that proper breathing, deep breathing, is a good first step toward a calmer, more centered, less-stressed-out you. "It's the easiest, most portable way to relax in the world," says Bette Jean Rosenhagen.

Before you practice conscious breathing, take a minute to read these tips. Yes, yes, we know that you know how to breathe. But there's breathing to keep you alive, and then there's breathing to enhance your life. *That* kind of breathing requires a slightly different technique. Here's how to do it:

- Imagine that your stomach is a balloon. With each breath you take in, the balloon should inflate. When you breathe out, it deflates. (Put your hands on your stomach, if you're not certain, and you can feel your stomach rise and fall.)
- Try to breathe in a slow, deep, rhythmic manner. If you want, you can count to three on each inhalation (in other words, one full intake of breath should take three seconds). Hold for a count of three, then exhale fully, again to a count of three.
- When you exhale, try to feel all the tension in your body being expelled

and released through that breath. After a few deep breaths, you can even try adding a word to yourself—"focus" or "calm"—as you exhale.

- Be aware of the breath, of the relaxing yet energizing effect it has on you. Becoming aware or "mindful" of this most basic of all human functions is the first step toward reducing stress. Once you do, you'll realize that this—our breath—is the first place we "hold on" to stress. We take short, rapid, shallow breaths. Regular, deep breathing helps us to let go of that stress.

This most basic exercise in stress management can be performed almost anywhere, anytime. "Just three deep breaths in the morning can make a difference in your day," says Bette Jean. Try it. Right now. Breathe in, breathe out. Slowly. Three times. Next, we recommend trying to carve out a few minutes every other day, even just five minutes. If you prefer, you can do it for longer periods of time, but you can still get the stress-reducing, anxiety-reducing benefits in just a few minutes a few times a week.

One last thing, if you're a perfectionist type: Be gentle on yourself here. As Bette Jean says, "We sometimes see people get stressed out over making sure they do the stress management techniques correctly." Deep breathing and the subsequent techniques related to it are not competitions. Don't grade yourself on this. Just try to let the simple act of deep breathing exert its gentle power over you.

So let's begin. You don't need special clothes, a mat, or a gym full of equipment to do this. You can simply put down this book, turn down the lights if you like, and sit straight in your chair, feet flat on the floor. Close your eyes and take a deep, full breath.

STEP 2: PROGRESSIVE MUSCLE RELAXATION

After a week or two of your regular deep breathing exercises, you'll be ready to move on to PMR, progressive muscle relaxation, a technique that feels a lot better than it sounds. You'll need a little more time for this, but it's worth every stress-busting second.

Sit in a comfortable chair, with your feet flat on the floor. Feel them touch the floor, make sure they are relaxed, wiggle your toes. Feel those toes on your left foot, all five of them. Now tense them up—yes, tense; make them *tight*, feel those muscles contracting, hold it for about five seconds and then . . . let it go! Let all the tension out of every muscle fiber in your foot. Feel your entire foot relax, totally, as the tension dissipates.

That's the principle of progressive muscle relaxation. Focus on a specific part of your body, starting with your left foot, then tense it up, hold it, hold it, then . . . whoosh. Let the tension out. (Make sure you continue to breathe normally during each of these movements.)

Move on to your right foot and head north, to your ankles, then your legs (one at a time). Be aware of your knees as they join your lower leg to your upper leg. Now move up slowly from your knee to your hips, glutes, and pelvis. When you get to your abdomen, pause and focus on the rising and lowering of your diaphragm. Stay here for at least two minutes as you refocus your attention on your breathing. Now it's time to move on to your hands. Make sure they are completely flat on your lap or on the armrest of your chair. Now, gradually move up to your wrists (one at a time), then onto your elbows, always being aware of those joints that connect one part of your body to another. Then it's on to Stress Central: the neck, shoulders, and back, where most of our daily tensions build up. Focus on the upper and outermost portion of the shoulders. Drop your shoulders as you exhale deeply. Now move up to your neck, letting your shoulders down. Very gently move your right ear to your right shoulder, then repeat with your left ear to left shoulder. Hold each position for ten seconds. Drop your chin to your chest, hold ten seconds, and then drop your head toward your back for another ten seconds. Feel the tension dissipate; feel your body totally relaxed, like a wet noodle.

There's your progressive muscle relaxation road map. It sounds like a long way, but as you tense and relax each part of the body, you'll feel a wave of calmness and tranquility moving up from toe to head. It's worth doing once a week. Think of it as a goodwill tour of your own body.

STEP 3: POSITIVE MENTAL IMAGERY

The great Flemish, Dutch, and German painters of the Renaissance can teach us a great deal about mental imagery. They went to Venice, studied with the master painters there, and then, when they returned home to Brussels or Amsterdam, they were able to re-create the brilliant light of Venice in their paintings. How did they do it? By "painting" a picture in their mind, a picture of Venice in all its shimmering magnificence. Through this mental imagery they could make the light jump off the canvas.

Are you ready for a little trip to Venice? Though we highly recommend it, the FORCE program can't book your tickets. But we can help you harness the power of the great Renaissance masters so that you can create your own light-splashed landscape in the comfort of your own living room.

We begin, again, with our breathing exercises. Plan to take fifteen uninterrupted minutes to follow this imagery exercise:

Sit comfortably. Inhale . . . exhale. Feel the breath pass through your lips, into your diaphragm. Feel the "balloon" inflate and then deflate. Do this deep breathing, which you should be comfortable with now, for a few minutes. Then, instead of focusing on the breath (as you've been doing) or on your focusing word when you exhale, keep your eyes closed, and let your mind wander to one of the most pleasant memories you have, the most beautiful places you've been to, the most wondrous sights and sounds you've seen or heard. Travel back on your honeymoon to Hawaii, to the day your first child was born; tune yourself in to the sounds of Mozart. Revisit a warm childhood memory or a special place you used to go to as a kid. Stand in awe in front of Michelangelo's *David*, or jump for joy as you win the lottery. Put yourself on a sun-splashed beach, beside a surging waterfall, or in the midst of a lush green meadow. Use all your senses. If your image is a beach, listen to the waves lapping the shore, the cries of the seagulls. Feel the cool ocean breeze in your face, and the sand in your toes. Look up at the sky, look out at the horizon.

Bring yourself home gradually. Breathe deeply, open your eyes, and savor the warm feeling you should have.

Visualization and imagery take practice. Listening to a tape while you meditate can help. Later, we'll give you some tips on how to create your own tape.

You should plan to visualize for five to ten minutes every other day to start. Eventually, you should try to do it every day. Visualize the positive places you want to visit; give yourself the gift of positive images that will help to keep the negative images at bay. Some who meditate or visualize say that the experience is like coming home. We like to think that it's also like going away to a very wonderful, warm place, like going on a trip that, when you arrive at your destination, feels like you're home.

Just as travel takes time, so will your ability to "arrive" at this relaxing place in your mind. Once you get there, you'll need a little time to unwind, to get into the vacation mode, just as we need a couple of days to do so on a real vacation.

Take your time arriving at the place of your dreams. Don't sprint to your destination; you need to ease into it. Also, try to make your image as detailed as possible. The more vivid the image, the better this exercise will work. The fifteen minutes you spend here should feel like an eternity. But don't focus on the time; don't look at your watch to make sure you spent your "allotted" time in paradise. That defeats the purpose of this exercise, which is to put some distance between you and your negative stress.

The value of positive self-imagery is that you guide yourself to a relaxed state, whenever and however you want. The beauty of the mental journey that gets you there is that you don't need to wait on a tarmac or buy a ticket. You can paint your own masterpiece, in your mind, any time you want.

MEDITATION FLIGHT PLAN

Most meditation or guided imagery instructors will permit you to tape-record their sessions so you can practice these techniques at home. Other students of meditation buy commercially available "deep relaxation" tapes. You can do this or you can develop your own mediation tape as part of the home FORCE program. Here's how:

Start with the goal of creating a five- to ten-minute tape. That may sound like a long time to talk into a tape recorder, but remember: Your spoken words are intermittent on the tape and are designed basically to prompt you and keep you focused on your meditation. The rest of the time is silence. (When you play back the tape, those silences will be the points when you should be meditating or taking your mental trip.)

Using a slow but deliberate voice, start off by reminding yourself to turn the lights down, close the shades or blinds, and turn your telephone ringer off. Remind yourself to eliminate distractions. Next, give yourself the basic instructions on how to get into the meditative state: "Sit down in a comfortable chair that has armrests. Try to make sure your back is straight and don't slouch. Keep your feet flat on the floor, arms on the armrests, and hands flat on your thighs." Remind yourself to loosen clothes, belts, shoelaces, and watches.

And now say these words, or something similar, into your tape recorder:

"Next, close your eyes, take a deep breath, and relax. Inhale, exhale. Feel your belly rise up with each breath you take in, and lower when you breathe out. Stay focused on your breathing. Breathe in, breathe out. With each breath you exhale, feel your muscles gradually relaxing."

Now, let's go through the body scan. Speaking slowly, tell yourself this:

"Focus your awareness on your toes and relax. On your heels, and relax. Your ankles, and relax. Gradually, work your way up to your shins, and re-lax. Go up to your calves and thighs, hamstrings, and relax. Relax your but-tocks, relax your pelvis. Let your waist relax. Soften your belly, relax your chest, relax your shoulders, relax your neck, relax your upper and lower back muscles. Feel all that tension in your lower back melt away. Bring your attention to your hands and relax them. To your arms, and relax. Relax your neck, your chin, unclench your jaw, relax your forehead. Breathe in and out and feel your entire body at rest."

The purpose of this is to bring awareness to your whole body and, obviously, to help it relax.

Now, give yourself two minutes on the tape to ease into your meditation. When you actually perform your meditation, your mind will probably start to wander at this point and you'll need some help to get back on track. Try speaking these words:

"Keep your focus on your body and your breath. Breathe in . . . and out. If any thought other than your breath appears, don't fight it. Instead, put that thought on a cloud and let it drift away, and gently focus on your breathing again."

Same thing if you hear a noise in the background. Tell yourself on tape:

"If you hear a noise, acknowledge it, then let it go and go back to your breathing."

After another minute or two, remind yourself to focus on your breathing. Conclude your tape by saying:

"Take two gentle, deep breaths and gradually open your eyes. Take as much time as you like."

You may feel relaxed when you conclude your very first meditation session, or it may take you a couple of sessions. Be patient with yourself, because with any new activity, there is always a learning curve. Over time and with practice you will become quite proficient in these techniques, but for now set realistic goals, such as visualizing or meditating for five to ten minutes four times per week. Eventually, you'll find yourself meditating for thirty minutes or more.

STRESS-BUSTING DRILLS

Ideally, we recommend that you practice your deep breathing three times a week and progressive muscle relaxation and positive self-imagery once a week. But there are going to be times, we know, when it's hard to fit this in. There are also times when you'll need it . . . badly. So here are a couple of ways to get the benefits of our stress management techniques when you have the least amount of time, or the greatest need.

THE NIGHT CAP

The tensions of the day sometimes build to a boiling point at the very time when we're supposed to be unwinding. Going to bed with a body and mind full of stress and tension is often why we can't sleep: we're all tensed up. Instead of pouring yourself a cocktail, take some deep breaths. Before you go to bed, sit on a comfy chair and focus on your breathing or your visualization. Ten to twenty minutes are ideal here, as it will put you in a good frame of mind for a good night's sleep. Allow your mind to drift off to wherever it wants to go during your Night Cap. If negative thoughts come up, acknowledge them, and then return the focus to your breathing. Remember: No distractions, lights down low, no phone, no television, and, if you do this drill correctly, no sleepless night.

THE TWO-MINUTE DRILL

In football, the pace of the game always gets frantic in the last two minutes. This is white-knuckle time for the fans, high-pressure time for the players and coaches. You need to think of your Two-Minute Drill as the exact opposite: an opportunity to slow down the game and reduce the frantic pace of your life for just a couple of minutes.

Football teams usually have a special plan in place for those last two minutes. Your plan should be to get yourself in a place where you can take two minutes to escape the pressures of the moment. Ideally, do this on your morning or evening commute—on the bus or the train, or even while you warm up your car. Another wonderful time to do it is on a walk in the fresh air (as we'll discuss in the next chapter, physical exercise itself is a potent stress reliever). But you can do the FORCE Two-Minute Drill anywhere, simply by closing the door to your office, or even by escaping into a bathroom stall if you have to! Just turn down the ringer on your phone, log off your computer, turn down the lights, and do two minutes of deep breathing. Sit with your feet flat on the floor, keep your eyes closed, and let those good, deep breaths do their thing. Exhale the tension; inhale the composure, the poise, and the perspective that will help you face the day's challenges.

THE DAILY HUG

We've saved the simplest stress-busting exercise for last: the power of the hug. Yes, the hug. Dr. Fran and other medical authorities believe in it—and with good reason.

"Hugs are a routine thing for me," says Fran. "It's part of how I practice medicine. I'm convinced human touch can turn out to be a source of healing for patients. It gives them power and strength. Don't ask me the mechanism by which a hug works. I don't know that we even need to figure it out."

Dr. Fran compares the power of a hug to a booster shot, bolstering feelings of confidence and caring and love. Touching, stroking, caressing, holding hands, cradling, putting an arm around shoulders—however you and your loved ones choose to express it, this loving, physical contact nurtures the spirit and improves health. And if you're not near any loved ones you can reach out and physically touch, consider this: some studies show that even cuddling with a pet can lead to a sense of well-being and reduction in stress.

THE POWER OF FAITH . . . AND FRIENDS

Many people find their stress reduction through their spirituality. This may mean a deeper exploration of your religion or a philosophical attempt to understand your place in nature. But sometimes, support can come from less obvious sources, from something as simple as a softball or bowling team. Participation in an activity and relief from social isolation just needs to become, for a while at least, part of your routine. The group is more than a distraction; it can also help provide stability at a time when other aspects of your life seem uncertain and turbulent.

You may want to join a local support group for patients with cancer (some of the larger regional support organizations include Wellness Community, Cancer Care, and Gilda's Club). Several studies have shown the value of such groups in enhancing quality of life and helping patients cope with their disease.

CHAPTER FIVE

EXERCISE AND PHYSICAL ACTIVITY

A diagnosis of cancer is a pivotal point in your life. It can force you to collect yourself, make choices, and take charge. It can motivate you to improve your health, maximize your quality of life, to be happier and stronger and smarter. You can use the illness as a springboard into the future. And exercise is the best way to help yourself.

Admittedly, few cancer specialists today share our enthusiasm for including regular exercise in a treatment program. But Dr. Fran, for one, thinks that's going to change, as more and more of her colleagues begin to recognize the value of regular exercise for their patients—and for themselves.

In fact, the Surgeon General has told us that Americans in general need to change our sedentary lifestyle and exercise at least thirty minutes a day.

The hazards of that lifestyle are well documented. If your doctor seems to question the efficacy of the FORCE program, remind him or her that numerous studies have been published showing that exercise can reduce the risk of developing cancers of the breast, bowel, and prostate, three of the most prevalent cancers in our society.

For example, an important Norwegian study published in the *New England Journal of Medicine* in 1997 showed a 37 percent reduction in breast cancer risk among women who exercised regularly, even when other risk factors for cancer were taken into account. This is only one of many persuasive studies that suggest the preventive efficacy of exercise for common cancers. And it stands to reason that if exercise can help prevent disease, it can also help you heal.

If you've recently been diagnosed with cancer, exercise can help you withstand the treatment program better. A German study conducted with patients who had undergone high-dose chemotherapy and bone marrow transplantation showed a great improvement in hemoglobin (blood counts), less fatigue, and higher levels of muscle fitness when they followed a medically supervised treadmill program three times per day, five days per week.

In an article in the spring 1999 issue of the *Annals of Behavioral Medicine*, researchers from the University of Alberta examined twenty-four empirical studies on the role of physical exercise as an intervention following cancer diagnosis. They found that these studies "consistently demonstrated that physical exercise has a positive effect on quality of life, following cancer diagnosis, including physical and functional well-being (e.g., functional capacity, muscular strength, body composition, nausea, fatigue) and psychological and emotional well-being." That's an important new contribution to the medical literature on exercise and cancer, and it should influence other oncologists' thinking about it. Dr. Fran is convinced that all her patients should exercise while undergoing treatment. She recognizes that exercise is a powerful way to enhance physical and mental stamina and strength.

Exercise is also the cornerstone of the FORCE program. Again, we're not saying that exercise by itself will cure you, but it can lead to some significant improvements in the way you handle cancer treatment. Here's how.

EXERCISE REDUCES FATIGUE

At least 70 percent of patients undergoing chemotherapy, radiotherapy, or hormonal therapy have low energy on most days. About 30 percent develop a chronic fatigue problem that persists when the treatment is over. _Regular exercise will boost your energy levels and combat fatigue. It even counteracts insomnia._

EXERCISE IMPROVES
MUSCLE STRENGTH AND JOINT FLEXIBILITY

Many of the medications used in cancer treatment can reduce muscle tone and strength. But _regular exercise during cancer treatment can protect the muscles and improve functional capacity._ Because muscles are the shock absorbers for the bones, _exercise will help prevent skeletal problems,_ such as fractures. In addition, _exercise can help you overcome the stiffness of postchemotherapy rheumatism and neuropathy._

EXERCISE IMPROVES YOUR BLOOD COUNTS

Regular exercise raises red blood cell counts, combating anemia and fatigue. _It also raises levels of white blood corpuscles, which are important in fighting infection._ And one study actually demonstrated improvement in platelet counts with exercise.

EXERCISE IMPROVES YOUR MOOD

Everyone, cancer patient or not, can use a dose of endorphins, the pleasure-enhancing chemicals released by the brain when you exercise. Endorphins are the positive feedback from your body. They are believed to be responsible for the natural "high" that many regular exercisers feel, and that you can, too. You will also feel, as many do, a powerful sense of satisfaction and empowerment in achieving even small increments in strength and fitness.

LET'S GO! THE FORCE
EXERCISE PROGRAM

This fourteen- to twenty-week exercise program was designed by FORCE exercise physiologist John Buzzerio, a group fitness instructor certified by the American College of Sports Medicine and a specialist in the emerging area of exercise and cancer. Working with the rest of the FORCE team, Buzz has put together a program designed to increase your functional strength and aerobic capacity. That means that this program is designed to get you back to independent living, to the day-to-day activities you need and want to do. By the time you finish the program, chances are you'll be stronger and fitter—in several important ways—than you were even *before* your diagnosis. Research suggests that people who exercise regularly tend to sleep better, have more energy, and have a more positive outlook toward life. That includes people with cancer.

The program involves three types of movement: "lifestyle" activity; aerobic exercise, designed to improve the function of your cardiovascular system; and resistance training, which will increase your musculoskeletal strength. We also encourage you to stretch regularly after your exercise, to help keep your muscles flexible.

That may sound like a lot, but as you'll see, it's really not, especially at the beginning. This is a conservative program in which you start by doing whatever you can do, no matter how little, and then progress gradually. The program is divided into three phases that will ease you along the road to a structured fitness program. You may need or feel that you want to add an extra week during the first couple of phases, to make the progress even more gradual. That's fine. Exercise caution but, please, make sure you exercise, no matter how slowly at first.

BEFORE YOU START

Here are some others things we'll need you to do first and some considerations you need to keep in mind. (Note: These are general guidelines. Depending on the specific nature and stage of your disease, refer to our at-a-glance charts in Chapter Seven for other modifications.)

1. If you haven't done so already, make sure that you get your doctor's approval. There are some stages in your treatment when it might be best to wait before beginning a program like this.

2. Every individual embarking on an exercise program should recognize that he or she is just that: an individual. And general guidelines and protocols are just that: general. You may be able to do more than the next person, or a little less, depending on your age, your current condition, and the shape you were in at the time of your diagnosis. There may well be some things that work better for you or don't work for you at all. As every personal trainer who has ever put on sneakers has told his or her clients, "Listen to your body."

3. This program is designed for any person with cancer. However, there are some caveats depending on the site of your disease. (For a complete list of these modifications, based on specific forms of cancer, please see Chapter 7.) But *breast cancer patients should follow these modifications in the resistance program*:

   • First, don't perform the wall volleyball exercise—in which you hit an inflated balloon against a wall—using overhead strikes. Hit the balloon with an underhand motion. You shouldn't be raising your arms at a higher than 90-degree angle doing this exercise.

   • If you've had a mastectomy and lymph nodes removed, avoid doing the biceps curl and triceps extensions for at least ten weeks.

• In our Phase II exercises, we recommend shoulder presses. Breast cancer patients can do this exercise, too, but not with more than one pound of weight in each hand initially.

4. "Do your best," says Buzz, "but don't overdo it." It's important that you start slowly. If you feel fatigued, cut back. If something hurts, back off. Discomfort and a little soreness are to be expected, especially as you begin to challenge your muscles, but never push through pain.

5. To avoid injury, follow the 10 percent rule: Never increase the volume of your exercise by more than about 10 percent a week. In other words, if you walk for fifteen minutes three times this week—a total of forty-five minutes—don't walk more than a total of 50 minutes next week.

6. Find a time, find a friend. Studies have shown that people are more likely to stick with an exercise program if they do it at set times (as opposed to whenever the mood strikes them) and if they do it with a friend or partner. Having someone to exercise with is of obvious importance if you're still weak from your treatments, or if you have balance problems. But it's also a good rule of thumb for any new exerciser. It makes the whole process a little more enjoyable if you're sharing it with a friend or loved one.

7. Make sure you drink plenty of water before, during, and after your exercise, even in winter.

8. Finally, remember your objective. You are not trying to "cure" yourself with exercise or transform yourself into a hard-boiled aerobics instructor. Your goal is to get yourself back to working a full day, to have energy to play with your kids, to be able to go for a walk with your spouse and not be fatigued for the rest of the day. Even so, many FORCE patients have been surprised that after fourteen weeks they were in better physical shape than *before* they were diagnosed!

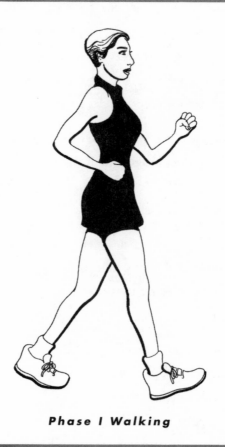

Phase I Walking

Oh yes, one more important thing: Have fun! Although fun is probably a concept that has all but disappeared from your vocabulary since your diagnosis, especially when you've been dealing with anything related to your cancer, activity and exercise can be fun. It can make you feel better, from head to toe.

PHASE I (4–6 WEEKS)

Monday and Friday: *Walking, 10–15 minutes*

Wednesday: *Resistance and flexibility training, seven exercises*

Tuesday, Thursday, Saturday, Sunday: *Rest (or routine lifestyle activities if you feel up to it)*

Phase I is meant to introduce you to exercise, to get your body back into a pattern of activity, gradually. You'll work on both types of exercise, aerobic and resistance, although you'll start off conservatively.

Our aerobic component begins with the most natural, enjoyable, and simple form of physical activity: walking. Start by doing whatever you can, without putting undue stress on yourself or getting yourself too fatigued. We recommend that to begin your program, you consider walking back and forth on your block, so that you can keep your residence in full view. That way, you won't have to worry about getting too far from home and then not having the energy to get back. We also suggest that you walk with someone. And in the event of inclement weather, you can walk up and down stairs. (Or, if you're fortunate enough to own a home treadmill, you can work out there. But be careful about using the treadmill at first, if you have balance problems.)

PACE, PROGRESSION, AND
PROPER PEDESTRIAN FOOTWEAR

Don't worry too much about how fast you're walking when you start out. Instead, focus on how long. But try to remember that this is walking for exercise; it's not a saunter or a window-shopping excursion. Former President Harry S. Truman (a famously consistent walker) used to advise people to walk as if they had someplace to get to. That means you should walk with a little spring in your step. Swing your arms, although not in an exaggerated, flailing, side-to-side style. A short, compact swing is better, your arms bent at 90-degree angles. Keep your head up, your back straight, and use a heel-toe stride. (A reminder again, that these are general guidelines. If you're walking right now with a cane or with assistance, *that's* how you start.)

What should you wear? A comfortable pair of walking shoes. Don't walk around in your slippers, in sandals, in high heels, or in those old beat-up shoes you use in the garden. On the other hand, we're not saying you have to go out and spend $100 on a state-of-the-art pair of shoes. And don't use the lack of a new pair of shoes as a reason to put off starting your program. Chances are, you've got a pair of shoes in your closet that are just fine to start with. As you pick up the pace and increase your duration, you can shop for walking shoes. Make sure they're flexible but offer support.

For the first week of your program, we recommend that you concentrate not on intensity or mileage, but on time. The goal for the first week will be to get you to walk for a total of ten minutes for each of your two sessions. (If you're stair climbing, which is more challenging than walking on a flat surface, walk for one minute, then rest for two minutes, up to a total of ten minutes.)

During week 2, try to increase the duration of your walk by two minutes. For week 3, pick it up an additional three minutes, to a total of fifteen minutes. And if you have to rest, no problem. "Rest breaks are not only permitted, they're strongly encouraged," says Buzz.

GET A LIFE(STYLE)

We talked earlier about the value of routine daily activities, aka "lifestyle" exercise. We've included it as an option on your weekends here. Why? Because we'd like to encourage you to start getting back into the garden, cleaning the house, waxing the car—the kinds of physical activities you used to do on a day-to-day basis but may have stopped since your diagnosis or treatment.

If you're not up to doing these activities in addition to the walking and resistance training, fine. But if you'd like to try to incorporate them, so much the better. Experts urge people to do about thirty minutes of these activities per day. Again, you'll be the judge, particularly at this phase of the program.

NEED A LIFT?

The answer is "Yes, you do." A lifting of weights, that is. The objective of weight or resistance training isn't to make you look like Mr. or Ms. Olympia, but simply to give you the strength to do the things that you love to do: basic, simple things like picking up your children or grandchildren, climbing stairs, or pulling yourself out of a tub. Our Phase I strength-training exercises require no equipment, and you don't need to go to a gym. You can do these exercises at home, using common household objects.

Cans of soup, vegetables, and fruit come in a variety of sizes, typically 16 oz (1 lb). Simple exercises can be performed by holding a 16-oz can of soup in each hand. To increase the resistance, multiple cans can be placed in a shopping bag or sack to perform a wider range of exercises.

If you want to invest a few dollars in some 5-, 10-, or 15-pound dumbbells, that's fine, too. You can either buy plastic-coated dumbbells of a fixed weight or you can buy them loosely by the pound and attach them to a small dumbbell bar. (When exercising, just make sure you choose a weight that you can handle for ten to fifteen repetitions or the number specified for that particular exercise.)

Always warm up before you begin to lift. A proper warmup consists of easy walking or movement for a couple of minutes. Also, remember to stretch afterward.

Follow the form as illustrated and described. Perform each repetition slowly and in a controlled way. A good rule of thumb for the resistance exercises is that the resistance (the weight you're lifting) should be raised to a count of two seconds, and lowered to a count of four. Also, please note that we've added some modifications on several of these exercises. If doing them the standard way is too taxing, consider the variation.

"These exercises are designed to strengthen your major muscle groups," says Buzz. "But just as important, we want you to strengthen your confidence and morale as well."

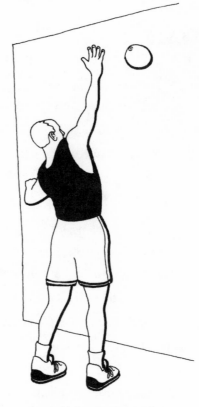

Wall Volleyball

STRETCHING AND RESISTANCE TRAINING EXERCISES

Wall Volleyball

Inflate a round balloon and stand approximately four feet away from a wall. Practice hitting the balloon against the wall using a combination of overhand and underhand strikes. You can make this exercise more challenging by stepping closer to the wall, striking the balloon harder, and inflating the balloon with more air. For added fun, try using a partner. This exercise concentrates on increasing range of motion and enhancing cardiovascular capacity. Perform this

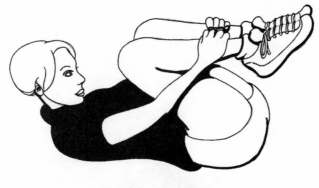

Double Knee Hugs

exercise initially for one to three minutes and gradually work on increasing your time. You can even use this as your warmup.

Double Knee Hugs

Lie flat on your back on the floor. Slowly bring both knees into your chest. Wrap your hands around your shins and bring your head up toward your knees. Slowly exhale on the way up. This is a safe and effective exercise designed to strengthen the abdominal area, as well as stretch out the lower back. Perform one set of five to ten repetitions. (*Modification:* Bring one knee up toward your chest, wrap one hand around your shin, and bring your head up.)

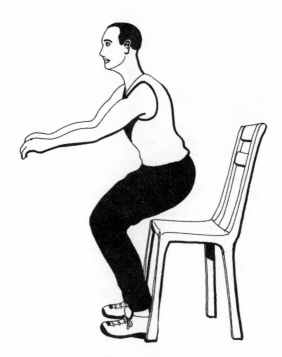

Chair Squats

Chair Squats

Place a chair firmly against a wall and slowly lower yourself, as if you're going to sit. As soon as your feel your buttocks begin to touch the chair, stand back up again. This is not only a terrific exercise that will strengthen your thighs, hamstrings, and buttocks, it is also a fantastic daily functional activity. Perform one set of five to ten repetitions. (*Modification:* If you have difficulty lifting yourself off the chair, use the armrests on the chair, a nearby table, or a partner's hand.)

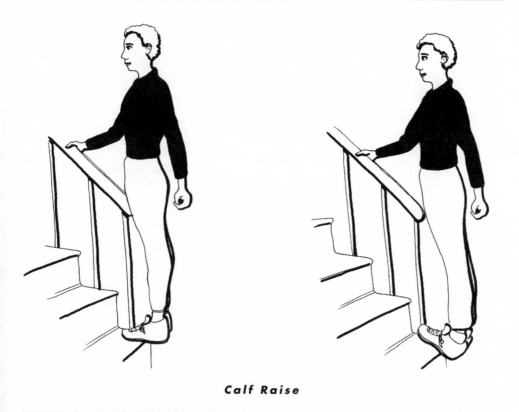

Calf Raise

Calf Raise

Stand on a staircase step, holding on to a banister railing for support (or use a telephone book placed on the floor and use the back of a chair for support). Place the balls of your feet on the edge, and slowly lower yourself to the point where you feel the stretch in your calf. Exhale on the way down. As you raise yourself up and onto your toes, inhale. Perform one set of five to ten repetitions. (*Modification:* If you have difficulty with this, simply perform the exercise on a flat surface.)

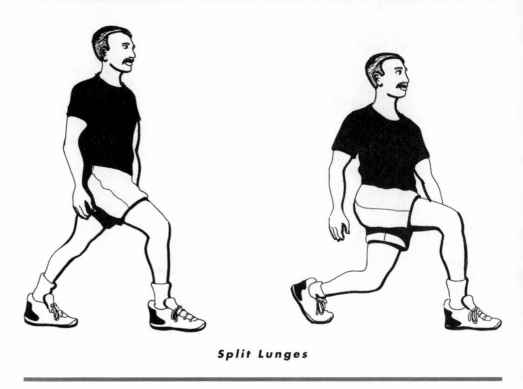

Split Lunges

Split Lunges

This modified version of a popular gym exercise is recommended by our friend and fellow exercise physiologist and author Liz Neporent. It's a great strengthener for the entire lower body. Start with your right foot about a stride length in front of the left. Then bend both knees, until your right thigh is parallel to the floor and your left thigh is perpendicular to the floor. Your left heel will lift off the floor. Push off the ball of your foot and step back into the starting position. Do the same with the opposite leg. (*Modification:* Don't be afraid to use a chair, table, or partner on this exercise, to help with your balance and to lift yourself up.) Perform one set of eight repetitions.

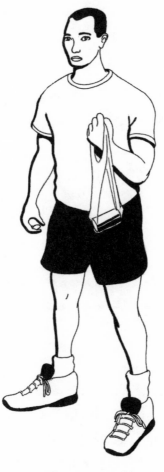

Biceps Curls

Biceps Curls

Place a 16-ounce can in a plastic bag with cut-out handles. Holding bag's handles as shown in the illustration, slowly bend your elbow up toward your chest. If you find that one can is too light, place two or three cans into a shopping bag. Exhale as you bend your elbow up, inhale on the way down. This exercise can be performed in a standing or seated position. Perform one set of ten to fifteen repetitions.

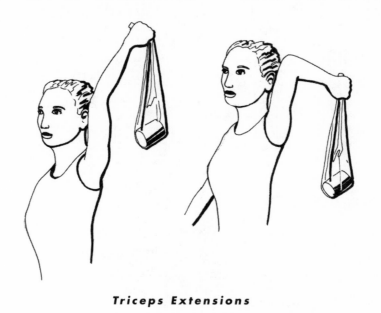

Triceps Extensions

Triceps Extensions

Holding the bag containing the can again, raise your arm over your head and slowly lower the can down toward the back of your head, making sure not to hit yourself. The only part of your arm that should be moving is your forearm. You may perform this exercise in a standing or seated position. Perform one set of ten to fifteen repetitions.

PHASE II (6–8 WEEKS)

Wednesday, Friday, Sunday: *Walking, 20–30 minutes*
Tuesday and Thursday: *Resistance training, 10 exercises*
Saturday and Monday: *Rest*

Phase I was your introduction, or reintroduction, to exercise. After three to four weeks of regular activity in that phase, you should start to feel the positive effects. You should be able to walk a little longer, and with a little more intensity. The resistance exercises of Phase I should be fairly easy for you now.

If you still feel you need more time, by all means, take it: add another week to the Phase I exercises before moving on. Then move on to the next phase in your own good time.

We've upped the ante a little bit in Phase II. Now you're walking three days a week (we recommend adding one day during the weekend, because that's usually when people have a little more time), and you're lifting twice a week. Also, we'd like you to pick up the pace now, and begin to focus a little more on the intensity of your walking. How do we do this? By using something called "rate of perceived exertion." This is a method of determining how hard you're working by using a scale from 1 to 20: 6 is very, very light intensity; 20 is the most intense, gut-wrenching effort. Shoot for 12 to 14 in your walking. Although everyone perceives exertion differently, there are some common responses. You should break a sweat at this level; you should feel that you're making a determined effort. On the other hand, you shouldn't be so out of breath that you can't talk with your walking partner. That's another good way to gauge intensity: If you can carry on a conversation while you walk, you're not working too hard. On the other hand, if you have enough breath to carry a tune—to sing more than a line or two of your favorite song—well, then, you're probably not working hard enough.

Along with the amount of exercise and the intensity, we'll ask you to increase the duration a little. Try to add two to five minutes per session over the first three weeks of Phase II. This will bring your total duration of actual time walked to twenty minutes.

Here are the Phase II strength exercises. Make sure you follow the same general guidelines about lifting that we discussed earlier.

Double Knee Hugs
See description in Phase I, page 71.

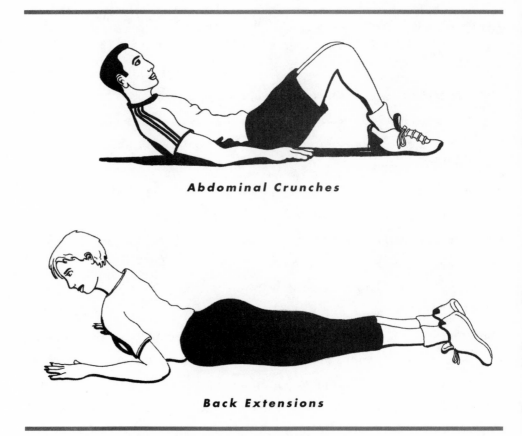

Abdominal Crunches

Back Extensions

Abdominal Crunches

Lie on the floor with your knees bent, your feet flat, and your arms on the floor. Exhale as you slowly raise your head—keeping your chin tucked—and your upper back off the floor. Your shoulder blades should never lose contact with the floor. Keep your head in line with your shoulders. Inhale as you return to the starting position. Perform one set of ten to fifteen repetitions.

Back Extensions

Lie facedown on the floor with your face turned to the side. Bend both arms and place your hands on either side of your head. Slowly raise your head and chest off the floor, keeping your hips down. Exhale on the way up and hold this po-

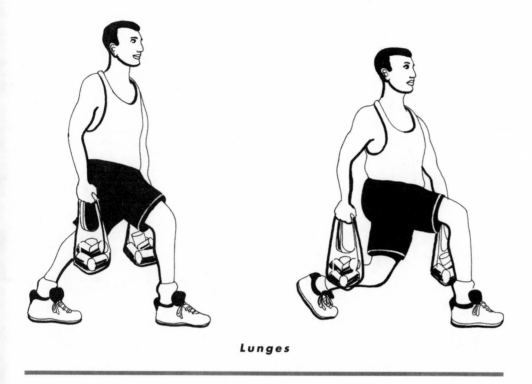

Lunges

sition for a count of two. Return to the starting position and inhale. Perform ten to fifteen repetitions.

Chair Squats
See description in Phase I, page 72.

Lunges
Holding a shopping bag in each hand filled with three to five 16-ounce cans in each, perform one set of ten to fifteen repetitions. If this weight is too light, increase the weight accordingly.

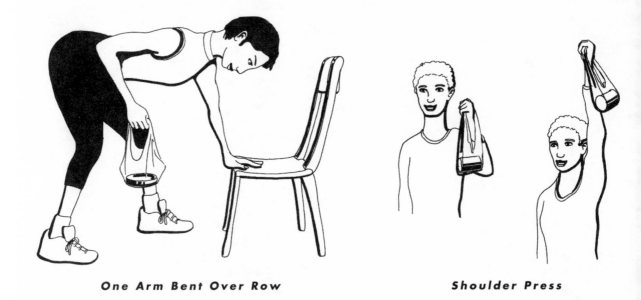

One Arm Bent Over Row

Shoulder Press

One Arm Bent Over Row

Fill your shopping bag with five to ten pounds of weight. Take the bag in your hand, bend over, and brace yourself with the other hand on a sturdy chair. Keeping your back flat (you should never perform this exercise if your back is hunched over) and keeping your head down, raise the bag slowly until your upper arm is parallel to the floor. Perform one set of ten to fifteen repetitions. Switch hands.

Shoulder Press

This exercise can be performed in a standing or seated position. While holding a 5-pound bag of sugar (or any weight that you feel comfortable with), raise your arm overhead until it is fully extended, then slowly lower until your fist is parallel to your ear. Perform one set of ten to fifteen repetitions with each arm.

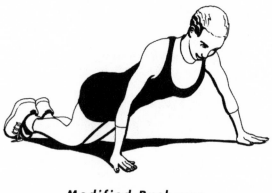

Modified Push-ups

Modified Push-ups

In this modified push-up, rest on your knees while pushing up. Exhale on the way up and inhale on the way down. Perform one set of three to five repetitions. If this is too easy, increase the number of repetitions as you see fit. As with all the other exercises, it should be challenging, but not too taxing.

Biceps Curls

See description in Phase I, page 75.

Triceps Extensions

See description in Phase I, page 76.

PHASE III (4–6 WEEKS)

Monday, Wednesday, Friday: *Resistance training, 12 exercises, followed by 30–45 minutes of cardiovascular exercise*

Phase III involves some significant changes. First, we'd like you to perform these weight training exercises in a health club, YMCA, YWCA, YMHA, or community fitness center.

Why a gym? Variety. More choices. More and different ways to get your body moving. Now instead of just walking, you can choose to walk or jog on a treadmill, pedal a stationary bike, or use one of the popular elliptical machines that give you a gliding, nonjarring, aerobic workout. Instead of using soup cans, you can use any number of weight training machines and choose from a variety of free weights as well.

Health clubs today are very affordable; you can even buy memberships for relatively short periods of time—six months, three months—and you can even join on a weekly basis or pay a day rate. For information on how to choose one near you, contact the International Health Racquet and Sportsclub Association (IHRSA) in Boston. See "Your Guide to Choosing a Quality Club," which shows you how to find the right, and reputable, club in your area. You can read it online at *www.healthclub.com* or you can send a stamped, self-addressed envelope to IHRSA, 263 Summer Street, Boston, MA 02210.

And, of course, there are alternatives to the health club: your local Y, for example. Many have top-shelf equipment and offerings that in some cases surpass health clubs, even though their membership costs are usually significantly less. In addition, many municipalities have facilities that may be available to you for a pittance. For instance, the City of New York Parks and Recreation Department has thirty-five recreation centers throughout the five boroughs of New York City that require residents to make a $10 to $25 donation per year to join. They have fitness rooms, gyms, pools, and tracks. Everything we recommend in this program can easily be done at such a center. There is probably something like this in or near your community. We suggest you check with your local parks and recreation department.

Another advantage of the health club—and some Ys and local gyms may offer this service, as well—is the availability of personal trainers. Once a luxury that only movie stars seemed able to afford, trainers are now a fixture in the gym, and, at rates that run from about $35 to $75 per hour, affordable. A trainer, even if you hire him or her for just a couple of sessions, can help make sure you follow proper form on the exercises and assist you as you make your way through the workout. The value of trainers was underscored in a study that appeared in the journal *Medicine & Science in Sports & Exercise* in the summer of 2000. The researchers found that subjects who were put on an individually supervised weight training program made strength gains at a rate 30 percent faster than those who were instructed as part of a group. So personal training can work.

If you decide to use a trainer, make sure you choose one who is certified, either by the American Council on Exercise, the American College of Sports Medicine, or the National Strength and Conditioning Association. Also, although it may sound like common sense, make sure it's someone you're comfortable working with. To find a qualified personal trainer in your area, contact the American Council on Exercise in San Diego. Call toll free (800) 825-3636, or visit the ACE Professional Registry at the organization's Web site: *www.acefitness.org*.

Another change in Phase III is that your training schedule now contains both resistance training and cardio work on the same day. One of the main reasons we make this shift is for efficiency. You may be getting back to work or to your regular routine now, so a combination workout is a better use of your time. Make sure you drink plenty of fluids and pace yourself. Of course, if you prefer, or if your schedule is better suited to breaking up the workout (that is, resistance training on Tuesday-Thursday-Saturday, and cardio on Wednesday-Friday-Sunday), fine. You can do any other combination that works for you, too, provided that you get three types of each workout done every week for these four weeks.

PHASE III CARDIOVASCULAR TRAINING: TAKE HEART!

Remember why you're in a gym setting in this phase: variety. Now is the time to start trying many of the different forms of aerobic exercise available to you: the treadmill, the elliptical machines, the recumbent stationary bikes. We'd like to suggest that, for your aerobic exercise in Phase III, you begin to use a slightly more precise measurement of your intensity: heart rate. To determine your target heart rate, simply subtract your age from 220. For example, if you're forty years of age, the formula is 220 minus 40, which equals 180. That number represents your age-predicted maximum heart rate. Our goal initially is never to exceed a heart rate of 70 percent of your maximum. At 40 percent of 180, our heart rate in this example is 72 beats per minute. At 70 percent of 180, our upper heart rate is 126 beats per minute. That's the range we're looking for. You should be exercising at an intensity that requires your heart to beat no fewer than 72 times and no more than 126 times per minute.

You can buy a heart rate monitor to do this for you. It's a great way to give you control over your cardiovascular workout. The monitor can be programmed for your upper and lower limits and will beep to let you know if you're working out too slowly or too hard. Indeed, heart rate monitor–based training has become very popular in recent years and many top endurance athletes use the monitor all the time.

But you don't have to use a monitor to check your heart rate. In fact, you can simply find your heart rate by placing your fingertips across the underside of your wrist closest to your thumb. Hold for fifteen seconds and multiply the number of pulses by four. Take your pulse at the middle of your workout—that way, you can make adjustments if you're working too hard or not hard enough—and at the end of your workout.

Finally, let's not forget this important caveat about heart rate training: The formula (40 to 70 percent of 220 minus your age) is a very general one, and varies greatly from individual to individual. The best way to determine your own target training zone is by getting a stress test (consult your physician).

PHASE III RESISTANCE PROGRAM

We've introduced some new movements here, as well as some new guidelines. If you are under fifty years of age, perform one set and keep your repetition range between eight and twelve. When you can comfortably and consistently perform more than twelve repetitions, increase the weight by 10 percent (which can be easily done by either raising the weight stack on a machine by one plate, or by adding small plates to a free weight movement). If you are over fifty years of age, perform one set and keep your repetition range between ten and fifteen. (This will ensure that you choose a slightly lighter weight, a wise precaution for an older body). Follow the same 10 percent rule here as well.

Remember: Proper form is the key in weight training. You're better off doing eight reps correctly than twelve reps with sloppy form.

One last point before we send you off to work: If you have any previously existing problems such as low back, shoulder, or knee pain, check with your doctor or physical rehabilitation specialist before starting to work on the machines we recommend. Those nagging problems don't necessarily preclude your doing strength training; there just may be some movements you'll need to avoid or substitute.

Though the machines recommended for these exercises are fixtures in most gyms, you may find yourself in a facility that doesn't have one or two of them. If that's the case, simply ask one of the staff to show you an alternative machine, one that works the same muscle group. And if you're ever confused about how to set up the machines, to adjust the seat height or leg length for full range of motion, don't hesitate to ask a staff member to help you. Improper settings on these machines can reduce the effectiveness of the exercise, and could even cause injuries. So make sure you're set up correctly before you begin.

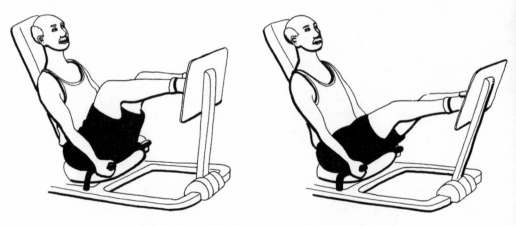

Horizontal Leg Press Machine

Warmup: 10 minutes

You can choose any cardiovascular activity for your active warmup: walk on the treadmill, pedal a stationary bike, try out the elliptical machine. Just remember to do it slowly. This is not the workout; it's the warmup before the workout. Also, remember that stretching, though beneficial, is not a warmup. If you have time, do some stretches now, after your warmup activity, and then again after the workout. If not, make sure you stretch after your workout.

Horizontal Leg Press Machine

Adjust the machine so that your knees are bent to a 90-degree angle. Keep your feet slightly wider than your shoulders, with feet turned slightly outward. Tighten your abdominal muscles so that the small of your back is flat on the pad (but don't hold your breath during the movement!). Make sure that your knees never go beyond your toes when the knees are bent. Exhale when you straighten your legs, but never "lock your knees," or hyperextend them when you straighten them. Inhale while lowering the weight.

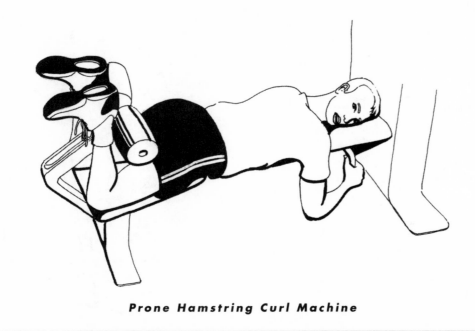

Prone Hamstring Curl Machine

Prone Hamstring Curl Machine

Lie on the pad, in what we'll call an "almost facedown" position: your face should be turned to the right (we don't want you mashing your nose on the pad!) and your chest flat on the pad. Position your knees so that they are slightly off the pad, with your knee joint in line with the axis of the machine (ask a qualified staff person in the gym to show this to you if you still have a question). Begin with your knees slightly bent and the weight plate a little higher from the stack. Exhale as you bend your knees up slightly beyond a 90-degree angle, while keeping your hips on the pad. Inhale as you slowly lower your legs down to the starting position.

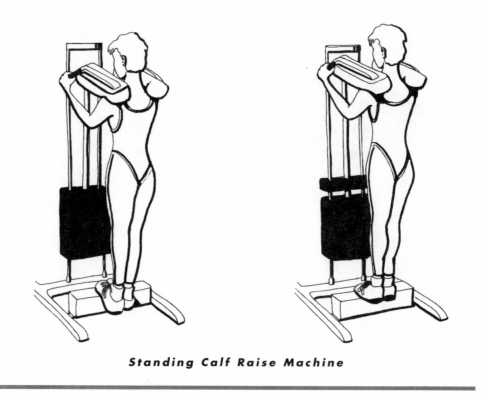

Standing Calf Raise Machine

Standing Calf Raise Machine

Stand with your feet pointed straight ahead, with the balls of your feet on the step and the heels off. Begin the exercise with your head straight, looking directly ahead. Exhale as you raise your body onto your toes. Inhale as you slowly lower your heels slightly past the step you have your feet on. Remember to keep your body straight throughout the entire exercise. At the completion of your last repetition, bend your knees while continuing to keep your upper torso straight until you feel the pad leaving your shoulders. This prevents undue stress on your lower back.

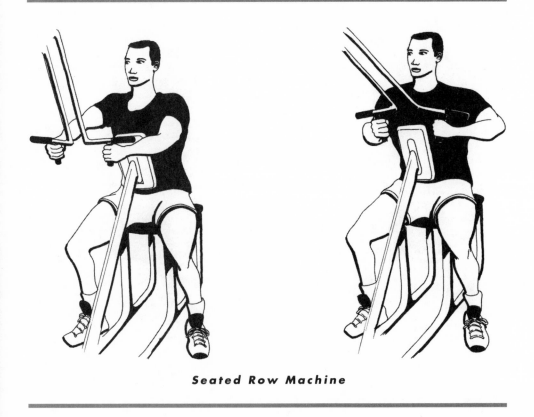

Seated Row Machine

Seated Row Machine

Adjust the chest pad so that your arms are fully extended when you take hold of the handles. Your seat should be raised to a height so that the horizontal handles are even with your shoulders and your forearms are parallel with the ground. Keep your head straight and squeeze your shoulder blades slightly together. Slowly pull the vertical handles toward your body. Exhale and continue to pull until your elbows are even with your shoulders. Inhale as you slowly return the handles to your starting position.

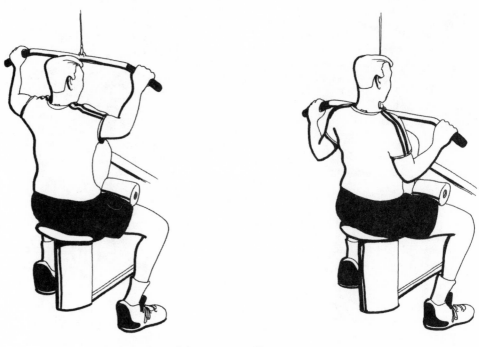

Seated Cable Lat Pull-Down Machine

Seated Cable Lat Pull-Down Machine

First, sit on the seat with your knees bent and your feet flat on the floor, and adjust the thigh pad so that you are seated snugly. Stand up to grasp the bar, placing your hands at slightly wider than shoulder width. Slowly sit down while holding the bar. You will be pulling the bar down to the front of your chest. Lean back slightly so that when you perform your repetitions, the bar doesn't hit you in the face. Do not pull the bar behind your neck! Lower your shoulder blades and squeeze them slightly together. Exhale and pull the bar down until your upper arm is approximately parallel with the floor. Inhale as you slowly raise your arms to the starting position.

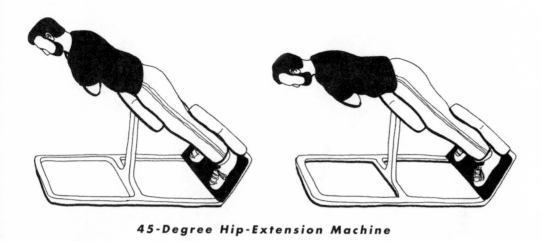

45-Degree Hip-Extension Machine

45-Degree Hip-Extension Machine

Adjust the hip pad so that it is slightly below the top of your hip. Keep your feet straight and your arms crossed on your chest. Exhale as you slowly lower your upper torso so that it is parallel with the ground. Keep your head straight without flexing your neck. Inhale as you slowly raise yourself back to the starting position.

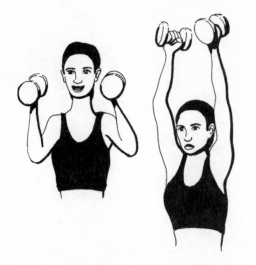

Standing Dumbbell Shoulder Press

Standing Dumbbell Shoulder Press

One of the best exercises for your shoulders. Start the movement by holding a pair of dumbbells at shoulder height, with the palms of your fist facing your ears. Slowly exhale as you press it overhead to full extension without locking your elbows. Inhale as you slowly lower the dumbbell to the starting position. You can alternate arms, or do them simultaneously.

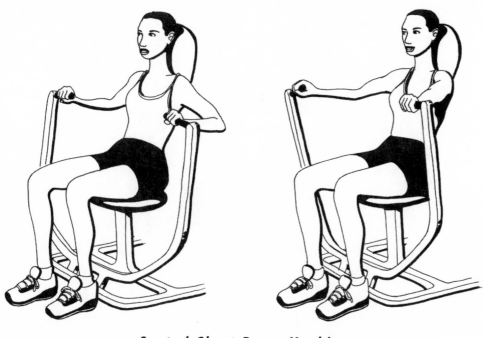

Seated Chest Press Machine

Seated Chest Press Machine

This is a terrific exercise to strengthen the chest area. Adjust the seat so that the horizontal handles are even with your chest muscle. Keep your feet flat on the floor, and slightly squeeze your shoulder blades together as you press (push out). Exhale—making sure you keep the back of your head against the pad behind you—as you slowly straighten your arms to full extension. Inhale as you bend your elbows until they are in line with your shoulders. Do not bring your elbows back past your shoulders, as this may place undue stress on your shoulders.

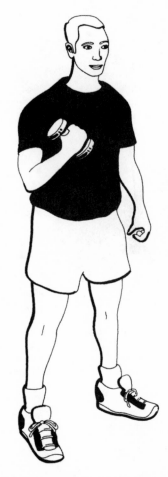

Standing Dumbbell Biceps Curl

Standing Dumbbell Biceps Curl

Stand with your feet approximately shoulder-width apart. Keep your head level, your shoulder blades slightly squeezed together, and your chin tucked in so that your ears are in line with your shoulders. Your knees should be slightly bent. Hold the dumbbells with the palms of your hands turned away from your body. Inhale as you slowly bend your elbow, raising the dumbbell up toward your body. Try not to move your elbow too much toward the front of your body. Ex-

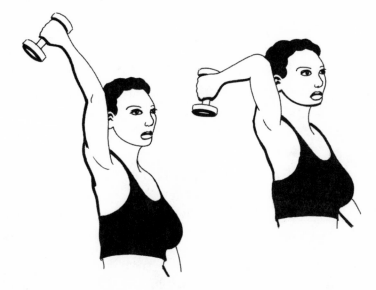

Standing One-Arm Dumbbell Triceps Extension

hale as you slowly lower the dumbbell back to the starting position. You can alternate arms, or do them simultaneously.

Standing One-Arm Dumbbell Triceps Extension
Stand with your feet approximately shoulder-width apart. Raise the dumbbell overhead with your thumb turned toward your head. Slightly squeeze your shoulder blades down. Exhale as you slowly lower the dumbbell toward the back of your head. Inhale as you slowly raise the dumbbell back to your starting position.

Abdominal Crunches
See description in Phase II, page 78.

Cool-Down
Perform your cool-down for at least ten minutes. This is a perfect time to stretch and to work on your muscle flexibility. For some, this may prove to be more

challenging than the resistance training because most people never stretch. The secret is to try to relax and to take slow deep breaths. Strive for a recovery heart rate of fewer than 100 beats per minute.

LET'S NOT GET
CARRIED AWAY, NOW . . .

The hardest part of any exercise program is getting started and sticking with it. By the time you reach Phase III of the FORCE exercise program, however, activity will have become a regular part of your life. This is just what we want; however, we also want you to be careful. Sometimes, new exercisers get a little too gung-ho and overdo it. Cancer patients, especially, need to monitor themselves for signs of overtraining. One of the best indicators of overtraining is your resting heart rate. If it rises ten or more beats above what it usually is at rest, for several days in a row, take a day or two off. Here are some other things to watch for:

- Insomnia
- Irritability
- Fatigue
- Loss of appetite
- Depression
- Decreased motivation to exercise
- Increased frequency of colds and influenza
- Increased frequency of injuries

MAINTENANCE PROGRAM

Congratulations! You have completed the basic fourteen- to twenty-week FORCE exercise program. You should be feeling some of the benefits by now: increased strength, greater stamina, more energy. You should be seeing some of the differences: firmer muscles, a little less flab. And most important, you should be feeling better about *yourself*—maybe not every moment of every day, but much of the time. That good feeling will translate into everything you do, your "quality of life." So how do you keep that quality high? How do you keep from losing the improvements and gains you've made? By sticking with the program, or, at least, a modified version of it. Here's how.

CARDIOVASCULAR PROGRAM

You've got two options here: fewer days, longer workouts; or more days, shorter workouts. If you do your cardio three times a week, shoot for forty minutes (and feel free to gradually build that up to sixty, if you can do so without undue stress). If your schedule allows for four days per week, you can do thirty-five minutes per session; five days per week, and reduce it to thirty minutes. It's probably not a good idea to perform cardio more than five days per week because you will require time to rest and recover. However, you can increase the duration of one session per week, if you like—up to sixty minutes per session—as long as you do so gradually.

RESISTANCE TRAINING

Use it or lose it. And you will lose it—"it" being the increased strength you've developed over the past few weeks—if you stop lifting. So keep pumping iron two to three days per week. You can either continue at the gym or go back to the exercises at home, using household objects or dumbbells. Either way, follow this general protocol: Do one set of eight to twelve repetitions if you are under fifty years of age, and ten to fifteen repetitions if you are over fifty. On those days where you are performing only resistance training, you may perform two to three sets. Rest at least two to three minutes between sets.

You can continue to follow the workout we used in Phase III, or you can mix and match a few of the exercises from Phases I and II. Or, if you continue at the gym, you can begin to experiment with other movements and different pieces of equipment. Again, make sure you learn and follow correct form. And don't go trying to impress anyone with how much you can lift (guys, this means you!). Follow these general training tips:

- Continue to check your heart rate at rest and during your exercise session. Doing so will help you monitor your susceptibility to overtraining as well as your intensity level.
- Do not let your heart rate rise above 75 percent of your age-predicted maximum heart rate, and do not let your rate of perceived exertion go above 14 to 15.
- Drink plenty of water before, during, and after exercise.
- Exercising should be a way of life. But like anything else in life, there is a tendency for boredom to set in. Vary your program every four to six weeks, choose from any number of the wonderful activities available, and, above all, have fun!

CHAPTER SIX

NUTRITION

E verybody seems to be talking about nutrition and its relationship to cancer these days, and with good reason. Research now suggests that dietary factors play a major role in the incidence of common forms of cancer.

Studies have shown that the population risks for common malignancies such as breast and bowel cancer can be altered by a change in diet. Here are some facts from the research: When Japanese women migrate to the United States and switch from the consumption of a low-fat, less-processed diet (the diet of their native country) to American society's high-processed, high-fat diet, their risk of breast cancer rises. Men who regularly consume tomato sauce (tomatoes contain the phytochemical lycopene) are more protected from prostate cancer. Hundreds of research studies have demonstrated a reduced incidence of cancers in people who consume more fruits and vegetables. Higher levels of vitamins A, C, D, and E, folic acid, selenium, and calcium have been associated with lower cancer risk. And drinking green tea, a lot of water, and less alcohol may reduce the risk of getting cancers of the bowel, esophagus, and bladder.

These and other findings suggest that what we should really be concerned about is our *overall* diet. But what our culture instead seems to be looking for is a "quick fix," a pill or a miracle food or elixir that will neutralize all carcinogens (and that will preferably come in several different flavors, chocolate included, and a super-size serving).

There is not—and there may never be—such a "super" food in the fight against cancer. But there is something that can help, something called a "good" diet. We can show you how to improve your eating habits and to incorporate many of the foods that can help in the fight against your disease. It's not as hard as you may think. Just as we recommend gradual changes and progression in exercise and stress management, we'd like you to approach your nutrition the same way: *Make changes gradually.*

The underlying principles of our FORCE diet are simple and few. We're not caught up in the "high protein" versus "high carbohydrate" battle. We eschew the fad diets, the extreme diets, the deprivation diets. Our program is based on some sound, proven principles and, we'll say it again, on *gradual* changes in your diet. You don't have to become a "food obsessive" or a nutritionist to follow this program. You will need to do some label reading, a little planning, and a little experimenting, but we guarantee you this: You'll still do some good eating!

FORCE DIET: BASICS

Our program is based on the experience of other nutrition and health professionals in the fight against cancer, as well as on the scientific research we cited earlier. We'll tell you why we make these recommendations and how you can incorporate them into your diet.

Implementing these changes all at once can be daunting to those who cherish their morning Danish, their lunchtime bologna on rye, their evening steak-and-potatoes. So we recommend that you do it gradually. Participants in the FORCE program are invited to make specific changes every week. You can do the same. For each of these five basic principles and recommendations, we'll offer a good "starter" tip, something you can do today to begin making the changes in your diet that can help in your fight against cancer.

TRIM THE FAT

Why?

Fat has been studied more thoroughly and linked more frequently to cancer than any other factor in our diets. But not *all* fats are implicated. *Saturated fats*—those found in fatty meats (beef, veal, pork, lamb), whole milk dairy products, and butter—are the real culprits. And these fats are sneaky: they even show up in the skin or dark meat of chicken and turkey. *Unsaturated fats,* on the other hand, come mainly from plants and fish. They also come in two types: *monounsaturated fats,* from olive oil, canola oil, avocados, and peanuts, and *polyunsaturated fats*, which include the *omega-6 fatty acids* from vegetable oils (such as corn and safflower oil) and the much talked about *omega-3 fatty acids* found in fish and flax seeds.

Heather Salomon, R.D., notes that recent studies have suggested that a high intake of fish oils (omega-3 fatty acids) may slow or prevent tumor growth, help chemotherapy drugs work more effectively, and reduce side effects during cancer treatment.

We don't mean to sound in*fat*uated with this topic, but there is one more type of bad fat that we should mention: *trans-fatty acids,* which are unsaturated fats that have been chemically modified to become "saturated." These seem to carry the same risks as saturated fats and are associated with cancer and heart disease. These fats are found mostly in margarine, processed snacks, and baked goods that list "partially hydrogenated oil" as an ingredient on the food label.

Bottom line on fat: Your goal should be to reduce the *total* fat in your diet to 30 percent or less of your total calories. You should limit saturated fats and omega-6 fatty acids while incorporating more omega-3 fatty acids for their potential protective effects.

How?

It's simple. Learn to read labels. Choose foods that have fewer than 3 grams of fat per serving (the government's definition of "low-fat"). Here are some other tips to cut the fat:

- Eliminate fried foods and fatty meats (hot dogs, dark meat poultry, marbled meats).
- Eliminate fatty foods (cream sauces, poultry skins, cream soups, nuts, chocolates, gravies).
- Limit consumption of red meat to no more than once a week or month, if at all.
- Be alert to "hidden" fats; for example, not all turkey burgers are created alike. Choose ground turkey breast, which has fewer than 3 grams per serving.
- Trim all visible fat before cooking.
- Keep olive oil in a spray bottle and use as a healthy substitute for cooking spray. Or you can use commercial cooking spray or a nonstick pan instead of oil.
- Grill, broil, roast, or poach fish and poultry.
- Choose tomato-based sauces and soups instead of cream varieties.

What to Do Today

Substitute one of the foods you regularly eat with a lower-fat alternative. If you're about to have lunch, choose turkey or chicken breast instead of roast beef or bologna. If it's dinnertime, don't fry your chicken—grill it. If you regularly eat at the salad bar, don't drown your lettuce with heavy, creamy dressing, and avoid the potato and macaroni salads. Just use vinegar instead, or put a little of your favorite dressing on the side and dip your fork into it *before* you start eating the salad.

If you're looking for a snack, put down the chips and instead pick up some raw fruit or vegetables or some low-fat, air-popped popcorn. Make a change like this at least once a week over the next seven weeks.

FIGHT CANCER WITH THE PHYTO-POWER OF FRUITS AND VEGETABLES

Why?

Dark leafy green vegetables; yellow, orange, and red vegetables; citrus fruits: think of them as a colorful, resplendent army—a rainbow coalition, if you will—in the war against cancer. The nutrients and compounds found in fruits and vegetables are powerful cancer-fighting agents for a number of reasons. Research suggests that these chemicals help the body destroy carcinogens before they damage cells, thereby reducing cancer risk. Also, fruits and vegetables are rich in the antioxidant vitamins A and C, which can help protect our bodies against free radicals, those nasty by-products of various natural metabolic processes that may have a role in causing cancer. Free radicals are also unleashed by smoking and car exhaust.

More recently, researchers have become interested in the *phyto* (meaning plant) chemicals found naturally in these colorful fruits and vegetables. For example, the *lycopenes* (responsible for the red color of tomatoes) have been associated with a reduced risk of certain cancers. The *organosulfur* compounds in garlic (see our section on medicinal herbs on pp. 120–124), onions, shallots, and leeks have been shown in some studies to prevent tumor cell growth. The familiar family of cruciferous vegetables—broccoli, cauliflower, and Brussels sprouts—contains *indoles* that may block carcinogens from entering body cells. The list of these phytochemicals and their role in cancer fighting goes on and on. According to our nutritionist, Heather Salomon, "There is much value in the 'synergy' of all of these compounds in the way they work together to fight all cancers."

How?

To get that synergy, Heather recommends a variety of fruits and vegetables: five servings per day to start, building up to nine servings a day in the long run. "We want variety," she says, "because no one food is a magic bullet, but a number of foods, working together, could have benefits." How do we do that? By creating a colorful plate! The greater the variety of nature's colors on your plate or in your salad bowl—from red peppers to green beans, oranges to blueberries—the better.

- Snack on fresh or dried fruits and raw veggies instead of cookies and cakes.
- When eating out, order a side of steamed vegetables or a mixed salad with dark greens along with your meal.
- To avoid extra fat and add more flavor, steam or cook vegetables in low-fat vegetable or chicken broth, and add herbs and spices.
- For more flavor, try sprinkling buttered granules, lemon, or vinegar on cooked vegetables.

What to Do Today

Try a new fruit or vegetable. Get out of the bananas-apples or peas-carrots rut and experiment with fresh, seasonal produce. There are so many delicious kinds that you've probably never tasted: papaya, mango, kiwi, star fruit, kale, Swiss chard, bok choi, for example. Tasted any of them recently? Now's the time!

FIBER UP!

Why?

Think of fiber as the Roto-Rooter of nutrition: it cleans you out by promoting the clearance of hormones and fats from the body via the gastrointestinal tract. But though our supermarkets abound in foods that would appear to be high in fiber—breads, cereals, and so forth—the truth is that many of them are not, because they're so "processed" and refined. The richest sources of fiber come from those foods that have undergone minimal or no processing, such as whole grain breads and cereals, legumes, and—once again—fruits and vegetables.

How?

Slowly—as in, slowly add fiber to your diet. We need about 25 to 35 grams per day. As the average American gets only 10, that means we should try to up the fiber significantly. But because introducing fiber-rich foods too quickly can cause gas, cramping, and bloating, we want you to do it carefully. Here's how:

- Eat a high-fiber breakfast. This is a good way to start your day and a good place to start adding fiber to your diet. Choose breakfast cereal with more than 3 to 5 grams of fiber, or mix your favorite low-fiber cereal with bran flakes.
- Choose cereals and pastas with "whole wheat" or "whole grain" as the first ingredient on the food label; choose breads with more than 2 grams of dietary fiber per slice.
- Like fruits and veggies, there are lots of grains not common to our usual diet that are excellent sources of fiber. Try brown rice, barley, couscous, bulgur, or whole wheat pasta in soups and casseroles or as a side dish.
- Eat more legumes: peas, beans, and lentils are delicious sources of fiber. Add them to main dishes, soups, and salads. Aim for a cup a day, because beans supply you with protein.

What to Do Today

Add some fiber to one of your meals. Choose bran flakes for breakfast. Ask for your lunchtime sandwich on whole wheat bread. Pick up one of those other grains at the supermarket and enjoy it as a side dish, or order brown rice and extra steamed vegetables with your Chinese takeout.

ADD SOY TO YOUR DIET
AS A HEALTHY SOURCE OF PROTEIN

Why?

Is there an Asian cooking secret we can learn from? Soytainly! (We always loved Curley of the Three Stooges and we couldn't resist a silly pun.) Some experts believe that the significantly lower incidence of certain cancers in Asian countries is largely due to a diet low in fat and high in vegetables and soy-based foods, such as tofu, tempeh, and soy milk. The phytochemicals found in soy are called *isoflavones*; they may help fight the development of hormone-sensitive tumors. In addition, soy components such as saponin, phytic acid, and lecithin act as antioxidants that may protect cells from the damage that can lead to tumor development.

How?

Try soy, even if you're not used to it. The good news is that soy can be easily added into your diet; in some cases, you'll find that it makes a very tasty addition. An initial goal on the FORCE program is to incorporate an average of one serving of soy per day, with an ultimate goal of 25 to 40 grams per day. Some tips on how to do it:

- Add cooked (canned or frozen) soybeans to salads, chili, and soups.
- Use fortified soy milk to replace milk in your coffee or tea or in recipes

for cooking or baking. Pour it over cereal, or use it as the basis of a milk-shake or smoothie.

- Tempeh—whole cooked soybeans fermented into a dense cake—is a delicious meat substitute. It can be grilled and added to salads or crumbled and used to replace ground beef in soups, casseroles, sauces, and chili.

- Tofu—soybean curd—may be the soy product best-known to Westerners. It's turning up in all kinds of dishes, perhaps because it takes on the flavor of whatever it's cooked with. You can add chunks of firm tofu to soups, stews, and stir-fries; you can use soft or silken tofu in dips, smoothies, shakes, or as the basis for soups and salad dressings; you can scramble tofu with vegetables and seasoning, mash it with bread crumbs, onions, and seasonings to create a tofu burger; or grill or steam it and serve with vegetables.

- Textured soy protein, which comes in dry granules, can be rehydrated with boiling water, and then used to add meatlike texture to casseroles, chili, burgers, and other favorites.

- So many meat and dairy alternatives made from soy products are now showing up on supermarket shelves. Soy cheese and soy-based burgers, for example, are among the most popular. Look for them; enjoy them. (We've tried many of these. They taste good!)

- Finally, the real soy-phobic can get it as a powder (isolated soy protein) in a health food store, and then mix it in everything from hot cereals and sauces to drinks and shakes. You won't even know it's there, but your body will, and it will use the phytochemicals to get healthy.

What to Do Today

Before you buy, try tofu: stop in a Japanese restaurant for lunch and order miso soup, which is usually served with chunks of tofu, or a tofu appetizer. Or visit your local Chinese restaurant, which usually has tofu (aka bean curd) in a number of its vegetable dishes. You could also stop by your local health food store or smoothie shop and ask for a soy milk or tofu-based shake or smoothie. Add it in gradually, because soy can disagree with some people. Still, given the various ways it can be used, almost everyone should be able to enjoy soy. Twenty years ago, only so-called health nuts ate it. Today, we know they weren't nuts, and healthful tofu and other soy-based products are much more readily available.

DRINK UP!

Why?

Water, of course, is essential to life, more so than any food. And we need to pay attention to what and how much we are drinking. In a mild climate with minimal physical activity, we require two and a half liters of fluid intake per day, 60 percent of which is derived from beverages. The body's need for water increases with exercise and climate temperature. Water is the universal solvent and is necessary for all the biochemical reactions of the body. Hydration is vital to the maintenance of blood pressure and circulation, the filtration of waste by the kidneys, and numerous other bodily functions, such as the production of tears and saliva.

How

Thirst cannot always be trusted to tell you if you need to drink more fluids. This is true for patients in cancer treatment as much as it for runners in a marathon. We need to tune in to other body cues. One of the most reliable is the color of your urine: if it's clear or very pale, you have been drinking enough water.

What to Do Today

Drink up! Instead of soda, pour yourself a glass of water to drink with your lunch or dinner.

A WORD ABOUT WEIGHT GAIN

American waistlines are growing rapidly, fueled by the current epidemic of supersize portions and calorie-dense, highly processed foods. And that's bad news in the fight against cancer, because obesity poses a risk for breast, uterine, colon, and kidney cancer. Research sponsored by the American Cancer Society and other organizations has attributed 30 to 50 percent of all cancer cases to an *over*supply of nutrients. Furthermore, weight gain during or after cancer therapy has been correlated with a higher risk of relapse, at least for breast cancer.

Don't get trapped by the old-fashioned viewpoint that cancer patients need to gain weight and therefore can wolf down whatever they want. And bear in mind that your treatment may be working against you. Treatment for breast cancer, for example, whether with chemotherapy or tamoxifen, has been associated with weight gain. So has treatment of lymphoma and prostate cancer. Fight back by eating smaller portions and by eating unprocessed whole foods that take longer to digest. Keep your total calories and fat intake low. (And, of course, start moving! Weight control is one of the many benefits of the exercise program we recommend as part of the FORCE program.)

Following the FORCE program diet and exercise recommendations should help you maintain a healthy weight.

LET'S EAT!

With these basic principles as your guide, you can now begin to steer your diet in a new and healthier direction. Of course, there are many more healthy foods than the ones mentioned above. To help you when you go shopping or plan your weekly menu, Table 6.1 lists Heather's suggestions of the foods to choose, and those to limit, when making your selections. In Table 6.2 you'll find a seven-day menu you can follow, plus healthful snack suggestions.

TABLE 6.1   THE FORCE NUTRITION PLAN:
THE BEST CHOICES TO MAKE

FOOD GROUP	FOODS TO CHOOSE	FOODS TO LIMIT
BREADS, CEREALS, RICE, AND PASTA* **(Eat 6–11 servings a day)** *Serving size* = 1 slice bread, ¾ cup ready-to-eat cereal, ½ cup cooked cereal, rice, or pasta, ½ bun, bagel, or English muffin	White, **wheat,** pumpernickel, rye, raisin, **multigrain,** Italian and French bread, pita, bagels, English muffins, hard rolls, flour tortillas, hamburger and hot dog buns Pasta, noodles, **whole wheat pasta, bulgur, kasha, millet, quinoa,** white rice, **brown rice, wild rice, barley, couscous,** cornmeal, **kamut, spelt** Low-fat** or fat-free **whole grain** crackers, flatbread, matzo, melba toast, rice cakes **Ready-to-eat cereals with 3g or more dietary fiber, less than 3g fat,** and low-fat cooked cereals	Breads prepared with eggs or cheese; fried tortilla shells Granola cereals Biscuits, croissants, muffins, doughnuts, waffles Snack crackers with more than 3g fat per serving
VEGETABLES **(Eat 3 or more servings a day)** *Serving size* = 1 cup raw leafy, ½ cup cooked or canned, ¾ cup juice	**Fresh, frozen,** or canned vegetables	Vegetables prepared with added fat, cream sauces, or cheese sauces

*Food items in **bold type** are your best food picks.
**A "low-fat" product has 3 grams or less total fat per serving.

FOOD GROUP	FOODS TO CHOOSE	FOODS TO LIMIT
FRUITS **(Eat 2 or more servings a day)** *Serving size* = 1 medium, ½ cup canned, ¾ cup juice, ¼ cup dried	All **fresh**, frozen, canned, or **dried** fruit Fruit juice	Coconut
MILK, YOGURT, AND CHEESE **(Eat 2–3 servings a day)** *Serving size* = 1 cup cow's milk, soy milk, or yogurt, 1½ oz natural cheese or soy cheese, 2 oz processed cheese	**Skim milk** and **1% milk** **Soy milk** and **flavored soy beverage (both enriched with calcium)** Low-fat or fat-free chocolate milk **Low-fat** and **fat-free cheese, soy cheese, and yogurt**	2% milk, whole milk, buttermilk, chocolate milk, cream All other regular and processed cheeses
MEAT, POULTRY, FISH, MEAT SUBSTITUTES, AND EGGS **(Eat 2–3 servings a day)** *Serving size* = 2–3 oz cooked fish, meat, or poultry, 2 eggs (4 egg whites), ½ egg substitute, 1 cup cooked beans, ½ cup (4 oz) tofu or tempeh, ¾–1 cup texturized soy protein, 3 oz soy burger, 1½ Tbsp isolated soy protein powder	**All white meat skinless poultry, lean ground chicken and turkey breast (99% fat-free),** chicken or turkey legs—no skin Beef, veal, pork, or lamb sirloin, beef and veal top round, and beef bottom round cuts Luncheon meats that are at least 95% fat-free **All legumes** **Egg whites, fat and cholesterol-free egg substitutes** **Soy protein isolate, textured soy (vegetable) protein,** tempeh	All other meats and poultry All fried, buttered, creamed poultry and fish Canned fish packed in oil All nuts and peanut butter Egg yolks Regular soyburgers and vegetable burgers All other frozen dinners

FOOD GROUP	FOODS TO CHOOSE	FOODS TO LIMIT
	All firm, soft, and **silken tofu** Low-fat frozen dinners, **soy burgers,** vegetable burgers	
FATS AND OILS (**Use sparingly**) *Serving size* = 1 Tsp oil, margarine, or butter, 1 Tbsp low-fat mayonnaise or regular salad dressing, 2 Tbsp low-fat salad dressing	**Vegetable sprays** **Olive, canola,** linseed, and **flaxseed** oil **Low-fat and fat-free sour cream, mayonnaise,** and **salad dressings**	Palm, palm kernel, coconut oil Butter, lard, cocoa butter, bacon or chicken fat Margarine or shortening made from hydrogenated or partially hydrogenated fats, or those in stick form Regular salad dressings and mayonnaise Regular sour cream, cream, and nondairy creamer
SWEETS AND SNACKS (**Use sparingly**) *Serving size* = varies	**Tomato-based soup, low-fat and fat-free soups and broths** **Air-popped popcorn, and low-fat butter popcorn** Sherbet, sorbet, fruit ice, gelatin, angel food cake, graham crackers, pretzels, low-fat baked chips, nonfat frozen desserts Hard candies, jelly beans, marshmallows	Regular chips (i.e., potato, corn, nacho) Buttered popcorn Candies made with butter, coconut, chocolate, or cream Cakes, cookies, pies, ice cream, chocolate

FOOD GROUP	FOODS TO CHOOSE	FOODS TO LIMIT
BEVERAGES **(Drink 8 servings of decaffeinated, nonalcoholic a day)** *Serving size* = 1 cup	**Water** **Dairy and soy beverages,** as above All fruit and vegetable juices, as above **Tea (black, green, herbal),** coffee, soda, other nondairy beverages	As above
CONDIMENTS	**Tomato sauce, salsa, BBQ sauce,** soy sauce, **chili sauce (meatless), ketchup** Honey, molasses, jam, jelly, syrup **Mustard, garlic, herbs, spices, vinegar, lemon juice, lime juice,** relish	Cream, cheese, or Bolognese sauce Gravies

TABLE 6.2 FORCE PROGRAM 7-DAY MEAL PLAN

Note: *Preferred beverages for all meals include water, tea, seltzer, coffee (no more than 2 cups decaffeinated beverages), orange, tomato, or prune juice (4–6 oz, although fresh fruit is better).*

DAY 1

Breakfast: Hot Cereal

1 cup hot oatmeal or cream of wheat mixed with 1 cup berries of choice and 1–2 tsps brown sugar

Lunch: Salad with Tuna

Large (colorful!) mixed salad: 2 cups dark lettuce mixed with ¼ cup shredded carrots, ½ sliced ripe tomato, ½ cup sliced red, orange, or yellow peppers and red onions (can substitute or change any of these vegetables for others), topped with ¼ cup kidney beans or black soybeans (canned, rinsed), 3 hard-boiled eggs (whites only), and 4 oz solid white tuna canned in water, drained, flaked. Top salad with fat-free* dressing of choice or balsamic vinegar. Serve with 6 whole wheat flatbread crackers.

* A "low-fat" product has fewer than 3 grams or less of total fat per serving. A "nonfat" or "fat-free" product has ½ gram or less of total fat per serving.

Dinner: Chicken Stir-Fry

Stir-fry ¾ cup yellow and red sliced peppers and ¼ cup chopped red onion in a skillet with cooking spray. Once onions appear glassy and peppers tender, add 4–6 oz sliced skinless, boneless chicken breast (previously pierced with a fork and marinated in low-sodium soy sauce for about 10–15 minutes) and stir-fry over high heat (about 3–5 minutes) until chicken is no longer pink and cooked through. Add 2–3 Tbsp hoisin sauce, 2 Tbsp low-sodium soy sauce, ½ cup pineapple chunks (canned in own juice), and 1–2 Tbsp peanuts (optional) to the mixture. Serve mixture over ½–1 cup cooked brown rice.

DAY 2

Breakfast: Egg White Omelet

Mix 3–5 egg whites (or ½–¾ cup egg substitute) with 1 Tbsp soy protein isolate powder. Cook with cooking spray and add 1 cup mixed (colorful!) vegetables of choice (spinach, tomato, red onion, green/yellow/orange peppers already sautéed for about 3–5 minutes with cooking spray). Serve with dark lettuce and tomato slices and 1 small baked potato (ketchup/salsa optional).

Lunch: Turkey Sandwich

2 slices toasted seven-grain bread with 1 Tbsp Dijon mustard, 4 oz fresh, sliced white meat turkey breast, 3–4 tomato slices and dark lettuce leaves. Serve with 1 ripe pear and 1 oz baked, low-fat potato or tortilla chips.

Dinner: Veggie/Soy Burger

Heat soy-based veggie burger according to package directions. Melt 1 slice low-fat American cheese or low-fat soy cheese on burger (optional) and serve on 1 whole grain hamburger bun with 1 Tbsp sweet relish, 1 Tbsp ketchup, lettuce, and tomato. Serve with potato coins and 1–2 Tbsp ketchup. Finish meal with fresh fruit of choice.

Potato coins: Cut 1 small baked potato into coins and spread onto a sprayed baking sheet.

Sprinkle with olive oil, garlic powder, and onion powder. Bake at 325°–350°F for 5–10 minutes, then flip coins and sprinkle olive oil and powders on other side and bake again until browned (for added flare, mix white and sweet potato coins).

DAY 3

Breakfast: Cold Cereal

1½ cup high-fiber (more than 3 grams fiber), low-fat cereal with 1 cup skim milk or calcium-fortified, low-fat soy milk. Sprinkle cereal with 1 Tbsp ground flax seeds and top with 1 cup sliced strawberries or peaches.

Lunch: Soup and Salad

1 can (about 2 cups) low-fat canned tomato-based vegetable, bean, or minestrone soup. Mix in 1 Tbsp soy protein isolate until dissolved. Add another ½–1 cup mixed cooked vegetables of choice (defrosted from frozen). Serve with 6 whole wheat crackers and a side salad with 1 cup mixed greens topped with ¼ cup unsweetened mandarin orange slices (canned, drained) and 1 Tbsp balsamic vinegar.

Dinner: Honey Mustard Salmon

Preheat oven to 350°F. Coat the top of a 4–6 oz salmon fillet with a thick coating of honey mustard and sprinkle with garlic powder, onion powder, and pepper to taste. Place on baking pan and pour white wine around the sides (about ⅓ to ½ way up) and bake for 10–15 minutes covered. Then remove cover, spoon sauce over fish, and broil for 1–2 minutes uncovered to brown mustard. Serve with 1 cup steamed spinach mixed with 1 Tbsp olive oil, 1 fresh, crushed garlic clove, and 1 baked sweet potato. Finish meal with 1 baked apple (core apple and place in bowl with small amount of water and sprinkle with cinnamon; microwave on high for 1–2 minutes).

DAY 4

Breakfast: Waffles

2 whole grain, low-fat waffles (heated from frozen) topped with ½ cup plain nonfat yogurt mixed with 1 Tbsp naturally sweetened fruit spread (optional) and 1 cup fresh berries. Sprinkle waffles with 1 Tbsp chopped walnuts (optional).

Lunch: Chinese Take-out

1 order steamed shrimp and tofu (aka bean curd on Chinese restaurant menus) with mixed vegetables (about 4–6 oz shrimp, 2–3 oz tofu with about 1–2 cups of vegetables), hoisin sauce on the side. Toss mixture in 2–3 Tbsp hoisin sauce. Serve with ½–1 cup brown rice. Finish meal with 1 large orange and 1 fortune cookie.

Dinner: Turkey and (Almost) All the Fixins

Heat 4–6 oz fresh turkey breast, sliced. Serve with ½ cup cranberry sauce, 1 cup cooked carrots, and 1 baked potato with skin topped with fat-free sour cream (optional). Serve with 1–2 cups mixed salad greens topped with 1 Tbsp chopped walnuts and 1–2 Tbsp balsamic vinegar. Finish meal with 4 oz fruit sorbet topped with ½ cup fresh berries.

DAY 5

Breakfast: Cottage Cheese and Fruit Platter

1–2 cups fresh melon cubes (cantaloupe, honeydew, pineapple,) topped with 1 cup low-fat, calcium-fortified cottage cheese and sprinkled with 1 Tbsp ground flax seed.

Lunch: Chicken Wrap

4–5 oz sliced grilled boneless, skinless chicken breast, ½ sliced red and yellow peppers, 3–4 spinach leaves, 1–2 Tbsp fat-free Italian dressing wrapped into 1 large whole wheat flour tortilla. Serve with 10 miniature carrots dipped in 1 Tbsp hummus. Finish meal with 1 fresh fruit of choice.

Dinner: Pasta Primavera

1½ cups cooked whole wheat pasta mixed with ½ cup rehydrated texturized soy protein (or crumbled firm tofu), ¼ cup shredded carrots, ½ cup chopped broccoli, ½ cup chopped mixed sweet peppers, 1 Tbsp oregano, and ¾ cup jar low-fat tomato sauce; salt and pepper to taste. Top pasta with 2 Tbsp Parmesan cheese. Finish meal with 1 cup decaf cappuccino with skim milk topped with cinnamon.

DAY 6

Breakfast: Scrambled Eggs

Mix 3–5 egg whites (or ½–¾ cup egg substitute) and scramble in a pan with cooking spray, with 1 cup mixed peppers and onions (already sautéed for about 3–5 minutes with cooking spray), 2–3 oz crumbled firm tofu, 1 oz slice low-fat cheese or soy cheese (optional), salt/pepper to taste. Serve with ½ pink grapefruit.

Lunch: Tuna Pita

Mix 4 oz white tuna fish (canned in water, drained) with onions and celery as desired, 1 Tbsp balsamic vinegar, and 1 Tbsp Dijon mustard. Stuff into one 6-inch whole wheat pita with 3 large tomato slices, 3 dark lettuce leaves, and 5 slices yellow bell pepper. Serve with a small side salad made with 1 cup mixed salad greens, 5 grape tomatoes, 1 Tbsp sliced almonds, and topped with balsamic vinegar.

Dinner: Chicken Fajitas

Sauté 1–2 cups mixed sliced onions and colored peppers in a skillet with cooking spray until onions are glassy and peppers tender but retain their color. Add 4–6 oz sliced boneless, skinless chicken breast previously pierced with a fork and marinated in mild salsa for 5–10 minutes. Sauté in skillet (about 3–5 minutes on high heat) until chicken is no longer pink and is cooked through. Mix in 1–2 Tbsp salsa to taste, heat and transfer chicken, onion, and pepper mixture onto separate plate. Heat two (6-inch) whole wheat flour tortillas and serve with ½ cup fat-free refried beans, chopped tomato, dark lettuce, and (optional) ¼ cup shredded low-fat cheese (or soy cheese). Fill each tortilla with combination of beans, chicken mixture, salsa, lettuce, tomato, and cheese. Wrap and enjoy! Finish meal with fresh fruit of choice.

DAY 7

Breakfast: Fruit Smoothie

Blend until smooth: 4 oz silken tofu, ½ medium–large banana (fresh or frozen), 6 oz unsweetened pineapple-orange juice, 2 Tbsp unsweetened crushed pineapple, 1–2 tsp honey.

Lunch: English Muffin Pizza

Two whole wheat English muffins, open-faced and toasted (4 halves) topped with ½ cup low-fat jar tomato sauce, ¼ cup chopped red onions, ½ cup broccoli flowerettes, ¼ cup mushrooms (canned, drained), ¼ cup chopped fresh tomato, and ½ cup shredded, low-fat mozzarella or low-fat mozzarella-flavored soy cheese. Heat until cheese melts.

Dinner: Sushi Take-out

1 order miso soup, 1 side salad with ginger dressing on the side (use 1 Tbsp of dressing), 2–3 sushi rolls of choice (6 pieces each). Dip in low-sodium soy sauce mixed with green mustard. Can add ginger to sushi. Finish meal with 1 cup fresh pineapple cubes.

Snacks

- Any fresh fruit (great choices: red grapefruit, oranges, all berries, pears, peaches, tangerines, melon cubes, pineapple cubes, mango)
- 3 cups air-popped popcorn
- Whole wheat crackers topped with peanut butter (about 1 Tbsp)
- 1 cup plain or fruit-flavored yogurt topped with ground flax seeds
- 1 cup mixed berries or melon cubes topped with 1 Tbsp sliced almonds or chopped walnuts
- Mixed raw veggies dipped in hummus or low-fat dip (made from dried vegetable soup mixed with fat-free sour cream and chilled)
- Whole wheat crackers with calcium-fortified cottage cheese
- 1 slice raisin toast topped with nonfat or low-fat cream cheese or calcium-fortified low-fat cottage cheese and sprinkled with cinnamon
- Baked apple with cinnamon
- Frozen banana
- Poached pear
- Dried apricots, dates, or figs
- Hot chocolate or decaf cappuccino made with skim milk

This is the diet we'd like you to follow. As you can see, it's based on the latest scientific research, not anecdotal evidence or somebody's intuition. It's steering you away from some of the foods that are harmful, and toward some of those that we know are beneficial. It will not cure your cancer—but then again, neither will many of the other, far more rigid or radical diets. We're not saying that vegetarian, macrobiotic, or some of the other popular diets are without value. In fact, our diet is largely plant- and grain-based and, like macrobiotics, does stress the importance of balance in the different types of food you eat. But making instantaneous, drastic changes as soon as you've been diagnosed—which many people do—is not consistent with the overall FORCE program philosophy, which stresses *gradual* change in your exercise habits, in managing your stress, and in working with your diet.

What this nutrition program *will* do is provide you with an eating program for life. This diet will help you feel better and stronger. It works in tandem with the exercise and stress management components of the FORCE program to give you new energy, psychological as well as physical energy, to battle your disease and get through the treatments. Most important, it will help you begin to regain the quality of life that so many cancer patients want.

You *can* feel good again. If you make these dietary changes gradually, within a few months you'll see and feel the difference. And you'll still enjoy eating!

Now, let's move on to some other aspects of nutrition that cancer patients often ask us about.

SUPPLEMENTS

Although an estimated eight of ten Americans use vitamin supplements (to the tune of an average household cost of $66 a year), scientific studies continue to show that virtually all nutrients necessary to good health can be obtained by eating a balanced diet of unrefined foods, the kind of diet we recommend to our FORCE program patients. Yet, people keep gobbling supplements like candy.

One problem in trying to get the truth about supplements is that the manufacturers and their products are not regulated by the government, and so are free to claim pretty much anything they like. And they make some pretty big claims about their supplements' ability to promote health, reduce weight, boost your immune system, or increase physical strength (without exercising, which is impossible). But buyer beware. And for you in particular, be aware of this important fact: No matter what promises or claims are made for vitamins and other dietary supplements, none has been proven to slow or reverse the growth or spread of cancers.

That said, we are not against supplements per se, just against the overuse of supplements and the outrageous claims of some supplement proponents. Taking a nutritional pill is *not* a substitute for good nutrition, but taking a daily multivitamin is a prudent habit. We know that supplementation along with a balanced diet is beneficial for certain populations, such as pregnant and breast-feeding women, individuals with a compromised immune system, children, athletes, and the frail elderly. FORCE nutritionist Douglas S. Kalman, M.S., R.D., actually recommends two daily multivitamins to FORCE patients who are going through chemo as a sort of insurance policy in case your body is not properly metabolizing food.

The vitamins and minerals that supplements contain are indeed important to your health and recovery, but the best way to get them and to get their benefits is through food, not pills.

MEDICINAL HERBS

For thousands of years, people in cultures around the world have used herbs—the seeds, leaves, roots, stems, or flowers of plants—as medicines. Today, herbs are gaining popularity in modern Western societies as more and more people turn to them as natural remedies, sometimes as an alternative form of medicine and sometimes as a complement to allopathic medicine. Surveys have shown that more than half of the U.S. population now uses herbal products.

We want you to be very careful about taking any herbal product when you are being treated for cancer. For example, you can go on the Internet right now and hear about some kind of herb reputed to "cure" cancer. *No herb can cure cancer.* But though we don't specifically recommend herbs as part of the FORCE program, we don't discount them, either. To help you begin to navigate your way through the thicket of traditional and alternative remedies, we asked Doug Kalman to review the five most popular herbs that have alleged cancer-fighting properties and to offer his pros and cons on each.

Before you begin taking them, talk with your physician. And make sure you have already embraced the three primary changes in your lifestyle: your exercise, your stress management, and your diet. These three practices will be absolutely key to your feeling better. The herbs' action will help only if you're already helping yourself. Make the modifications we've recommended *first*; then, you can begin to explore the following herbs to see if they make sense for you.

Remember that, like supplements, herbal products are not subject to regulation. Tests have shown that many products contain less of the active ingredients of the herb or less of the herb itself than promised on the label. Some may contain none at all; others are wildly overpriced. If you're going to buy these products, we recommend going to a reputable health food store.

ECHINACEA

What Is It?

Also known as purple coneflower, echinacea is a wildflower native to North America. It was used by Native Americans to treat wounds and respiratory infections and, since the late 1800s, has been used by the general population.

What Does It Do?

The primary value of echinacea is said to be its ability to increase resistance to infection. Extracts prepared from the roots and stems are said to "boost" the body's immune system. Many people today take echinacea to prevent or treat colds and the flu. The plant contains a number of active compounds that appear to stimulate the production and activity of white blood cells, whose function is to attack and destroy bacteria and other disease-causing invaders in the bloodstream. Echinacea may also increase production of cytokines, chemicals that help control immune system activity.

Will It Help Me?

Echinacea can be helpful in relieving colds and infections from bacteria, viruses, and yeast. It appears to have some effect on reducing inflammation. Research is under way to evaluate echinacea's potential role in treating serious diseases, including cancer. In some laboratory studies, echinacea was found to stimulate release of interleukins, interferon, and tumor necrosis factor, chemicals that may play a role in controlling the growth of cancerous cells. Other studies have not seen such results.

GARLIC

What Is It?

Garlic, a member of the onion family, has been used for thousands of years as both a food and an herbal remedy. The bulb contains a cluster of separate pieces, called cloves, enclosed in a papery skin.

What Does It Do?

Scientific studies confirm that garlic helps prevent atherosclerosis ("hardening of the arteries") by lowering cholesterol and triglyceride levels in the blood. It prevents the formation of blood clots by reducing the stickiness of platelets and by fibrinolysis (preventing clotting proteins from forming a mesh that can trap blood cells).

Will It Help Me?

Garlic extract, powders, or cloves can stimulate the immune system by triggering the proliferation of lymphocytes, boosting the release of cytokines, and promoting the activity of natural killer cells. But it's important to remember that you can consume adequate levels of garlic simply by increasing how much you eat in foods you prepare.

GINGER

What Is It?

Ginger is a perennial plant that grows in India, China, Mexico, and other regions. Its roots are used as a spice and an herbal remedy.

What Does It Do?

Ginger has been used in traditional Chinese and Indian medicine for thousands of years as a remedy for digestive problems, nausea and vomiting, cough, and inflammatory diseases.

Will It Help Me?

Research on the use of ginger as a treatment for cancer is under way. Experimental studies in mice show that curcumin, a compound found in ginger and related plants, inhibits the development of skin tumors and triggers the death of cancer cells. Pungent compounds may also work as antioxidants, thus reducing the risk of cell damage that can lead to cancer. Still, at this time, evidence does not show that ginger is effective in preventing or treating cancer in humans.

GINKGO BILOBA

What Is It?

Also known as the maidenhair tree, ginkgo is the oldest living species of tree on the planet. Ginkgo is common in China, where it was considered sacred and was used to decorate temple gardens. The leaves of the ginkgo are fan-shaped and have two distinct sections, or lobes (hence the term "biloba").

What Does It Do?

It is considered a remedy for respiratory ailments and is used commonly today as a treatment for memory loss in the elderly. Ginkgo acts as a blood thinner, so you should not take it if you need blood tests or surgery, as it reduces the blood's ability to clot.

Will It Help Me?

Research on the potential role of ginkgo as a cancer treatment is in its early stages. Laboratory studies suggest that some ginkgo compounds, known as phenols, may inhibit the growth of certain types of human tumors. Research in Russia on people who live near the site of the Chernobyl nuclear accident suggests that use of ginkgo, an antioxidant, may prevent damage to DNA (the genetic component of cells) that results from exposure to radiation. More research is needed before claims of efficacy against cancer can be made.

GINSENG

What Is It?

The name ginseng applies to a family of plants, of which there are about seven hundred species. Ginseng grows in tropical and temperate climates and is common in the Americas and Asia. The ginseng root is believed to possess many medical properties. There are two main types of ginseng available as an herbal remedy: Asian ginseng, also called Chinese or Korean ginseng, and Siberian ginseng, a distant relative of Asian ginseng also known as eleuthero, touch-me-not, and devil's shrub.

What Does It Do?

Chinese ginseng contains a number of compounds that are thought to act together to produce its beneficial effects. Siberian ginseng is used to prevent colds, flu, and respiratory tract infections. Some people claim it increases stamina and endurance.

Will It Help Me?

Despite the use of ginseng by people of many cultures for many years, the evidence that it is effective is largely anecdotal. A ginsenoside compound was found to increase the ability of a chemotherapy drug, cisplatin, in preventing the spread of ovarian cancer. A 1990 study from Korea found that people who took ginseng were less likely to develop cancer than those who did not. In this study, ginseng extract and powder were considered more effective than fresh sliced ginseng or ginseng juice or tea. Ginseng consumption in the diet also has been associated with a decreased risk of gastric cancer among people of South Korea.

CHAPTER SEVEN

EXERCISE AND MOVEMENT REGIMENS FOR SPECIFIC CANCERS

I n the main text of this book, we've provided a core program for men and women battling cancer. Here, in easy-to-read chart form, are disease-specific prescriptions for, as well as some basic facts about, six common forms of cancer.

BREAST CANCER

Outside of skin cancer, breast cancer is the most common type of cancer among women in the United States. Each year in this country, more than 180,000 women—and 1,000 men—are diagnosed with breast cancer.*

At the first meeting of the Athletes Support Group, the forerunner of the FORCE program, twenty people attended, half of them women. Of these ten women, nine had been diagnosed with breast cancer. These numbers hit home for the men in the group, and by the end of that first meeting they had a new understanding of just how vulnerable their own wives, mothers, daughters, sisters, and women friends were to this disease. At that meeting the group decided to devote a future session entirely to understanding breast cancer.

*The source of statistics in this chapter is the American Cancer Society.

Jeff decided to get more active in the fight against breast cancer. In 1997, he was named chair of Three Miles of Men, a group whose purpose was to support women participating in the New York City edition of the Race for the Cure, a 5K (3.1 mile) race designed to raise funds and awareness about breast cancer prevention and education. Three Miles of Men recruited spouses and friends to be spectators along the three-mile course of the race.

With or without the men, the Race for the Cure is a phenomenally successful event. This nationwide series, which benefits the Susan G. Komen Breast Cancer Foundation, has grown over the past decade to the point that it is now one of the dominant events in the sport of road running. In 1999, according to USA Track & Field Road Running Information Center in Santa Barbara, a total of 688,000 women crossed the finish line of at least one of the 107 Race for the Cure events held annually in the United States. The individual events themselves attract staggering numbers of participants. The largest Race for the Cure, held in Washington, D.C., had 46,060 finishers in 1999, making it the third largest race of any kind in the United States.

All of these women, whether walkers or runners, are concerned about breast cancer. Many are survivors themselves (they distinguish themselves by wearing pink ribbons, shirts, and hats—an inspiring sight); others run to honor the memories of loved ones lost to the disease; still others run or walk simply because it's a good cause.

The Susan G. Komen Breast Cancer Foundation, largely through the money raised through the races, has become the number-one funding organization for breast cancer research. By emphasizing activity and fitness, it epitomizes the spirit and principles of the FORCE program. The Race for the Cure invites women to vote with their feet, so to speak: to show that women with breast cancer can still be healthy and vital. Indeed, many of the women who have come through the FORCE program are breast cancer survivors, and many of them participate regularly in the local Race for the Cure. Chances are, there's one not far from you. If you're a woman, we encourage you to participate in it. Use it as the culmination of your three-phase exercise program. A 5K walk or run is a good workout, and of course, you'll be part of something much larger. If you're a guy, why not go out and support this effort? (For more information, visit *www.raceforthecure.com.*)

Now let's talk some more about exercise and breast cancer. If you have had a mastectomy or lumpectomy, you will undoubtedly be put on a postsurgical rehabilitation program, in which some form of exercise will be prescribed, depending on the stage and extent of the disease and the particular treatment you receive. Specific exercises after surgery can help to strengthen the affected area and will also help to reduce postsurgical pain and stiffness. In as little as a day or two following surgery, these exercises can begin under the guidance of a doctor, nurse, or physical therapist. The key is to be very slow and gentle in the beginning. Remember, many of these exercises are basic and designed to promote blood flow and help you to regain some strength and flexibility. Typically, they might involve simply walking your fingers up and down the wall or swinging your arms in a circle while holding a light weight.

You should do these exercises, of course, and follow the guidelines laid out by your cancer care providers, for the first four to six weeks following surgery. After that, and, as always, with your physician's approval, you should be ready to begin Phase I of the FORCE exercise program, as outlined in Chapter 5.

In that chapter, we listed some specific exercise modifications for breast cancer patients. We list some other modifications in Table 7.1 specific to your form of cancer and the kind of treatment you've received. But here's one more general suggestion about resistance training: In physical therapy—and, increasingly, in the general fitness arena, as well—elastic tubing is often used in resistance training. You can't gauge precisely how much you're lifting with tubing, as you can with free weights and machines (and the tube workouts are generally thought to be a little less challenging), but they are still a great way to build strength safely, especially in the weeks and months immediately after surgery. Another benefit is that you can work out at home.

If you'd like to incorporate or substitute some of our Phase I exercises with resistance bands or tube movements, feel free. If you belong to a gym, you can ask about the availability of classes or instructors who utilize these stretchable bands or tubes (they go by different brand names, including Dynabands and Exer-stretch). Or you can order it yourself. Two good sources are Spri Products (call 800-222-7774 for a catalogue) and the following Web site, devoted to the healing art of Reiki, which offers a catalogue of resistance tubing products, plus instructions and sample exercises: *www.reikihealingministry.com.*

PROSTATE CANCER

The prostate, which produces a fluid that forms part of the semen, is a walnut-sized gland located below the bladder and in front of the rectum. Aside from skin cancer, prostate cancer is the most common type of cancer in men in the United States.

A couple of years ago, Jeff spoke at a meeting of Us Too!, a national prostate cancer research and support organization, at Memorial Sloan-Kettering Cancer Center. He was shocked to find that more than two hundred men and women had filled the auditorium to hear about the latest research and surgical techniques affecting prostate cancer patients. "Many of these guys were in their sixties and full of vigor," he recalls. "They came with laptop computers, notepads,

TABLE 7.1   BREAST CANCER REGIMENS

TREATMENT	AEROBIC ACTIVITY	STRENGTH TRAINING	NUTRITIONAL SUPPORT
	(FORCE MODIFICATIONS)	(FORCE MODIFICATIONS)	
BREAST/ CHEMOTHERAPY/ RADIATION TREATMENT	Water aerobics (no swimming), treadmill walking, stationary bicycle throughout treatment cycle. First month after treatment begins, 2–3 times a week. Duration: 15–30 min.	Maintain stretching/ flexibility movements throughout entire treatment cycle. Utilize recommended stretches in Chapter 5. Stretch for 10–15 min a day, total body (2–4 times a week).	Lower saturated fat to less than 10%. Lower total fat to 20–25% of dietary intake. Maintain a high nutrient-rich diet.
	Incorporate up to 30 min a day 3–4 times a week aerobic exercises based on your personal preference. Avoid exercising on the day before, day of, and day after chemotherapy treatment.	During treatment for the first 4–8 weeks, begin weight-bearing activities with 2–5 lbs. Follow Phase I soup can workout in Chapter 5.	Increase intake of fruits and vegetables to 5–9 servings a day from 5 a day. Increase intake of folic acid found in asparagus, broccoli, legumes, and orange juice.

TREATMENT	AEROBIC ACTIVITY	STRENGTH TRAINING	NUTRITIONAL SUPPORT
BREAST/ CHEMOTHERAPY/ RADIATION TREATMENT CONT'D	Aerobic exercise should consist of an effort level of 50–70% of your maximum heart rate.	Incorporate use of flexible resistance bands and tubing for most forms of resistance training.	Include protein-rich foods other than red meats. Eat fish that is high in omega-3 fatty acids such as salmon, sea bass, or halibut.
	While undergoing intensive radiation therapy, maintain schedule as above. You may need to curtail your exercise in the latter stages of treatment due to cumulative side effects.	It's not necessary to increase the amount of weight you're training with during your radiation treatment, especially if it occurs simul-taneously with chemotherapy.	Take 1–2 multivitamins per day that include folic acid. During treatment, limit introducing new supplements and vitamins to your diet.
ESTROGEN POSITIVE	Above recommendations apply.	Above recommendations apply.	Limit soy intake.
BREAST/SURGERY MASTECTOMY/ LUMPECTOMY	Treadmill walking, stationary bicycle for first 6 weeks beginning at least 4 weeks postsurgery (2–3 times a week). If suffi-cient level of fit-ness exists prior to surgery,	Begin stretching/ flexibility movements 4–6 weeks after surgery utilizing recommended stretches in Chapter 5. Start with 5–10 min a day, total body	Lower saturated fat to less than 25% of dietary intake 4 weeks after surgery. Lower total fat to 30% of dietary intake.

TREATMENT	AEROBIC ACTIVITY	STRENGTH TRAINING	NUTRITIONAL SUPPORT
BREAST/SURGERY MASTECTOMY/ LUMPECTOMY CONT'D	with doctor's approval, may begin at 2 weeks (10–15 min per session).	(2–4 times a week). If stretching/ flexing prior to surgery, begin after 2–4 weeks.	
	Incorporate 20–30 min a day 3–4 times a week exercises based on your personal preference. Keep all aerobic exercises, whether inside or outside, in a well-defined area, such as a local track or your own neighborhood.	4–6 weeks after surgery, begin weight-bearing activities with no more than 5 lbs initially for your lower body only. After 6–8 weeks, you may begin weight-bearing exercises for your upper body with no more than 2–5 lbs (see Chap. 5 for Phase I recommendations).	Slowly increase your intake of fruits and vegetables. First build up to 5 servings per day and then increase your intake to 9 servings per day.
	Aerobic exercise should consist of an effort level of 70% of your maximum heart rate. Keep exercise to a maximum of 40 min no more than 4 days a week.	Incorporate the use of flexible resistance tubing or bands for most forms of resistance training. Target deltoid (shoulder), pectoral (chest), upper back, biceps, and triceps muscles.	Include protein-rich foods other than red meats. Include skinless white meat chicken and turkey along with increasing your intake of fish (sole, salmon, halibut, red snapper, tuna).

TREATMENT	AEROBIC ACTIVITY	STRENGTH TRAINING	NUTRITIONAL SUPPORT
BREAST/SURGERY MASTECTOMY/ LUMPECTOMY CONT'D	After 8–10 weeks establishing an aerobic base, slowly begin aerobic exercises unaided by the use of a treadmill or exercise bicycle. Avoid steep uphill and downhill grades.	For all upper-body weight-bearing exercises, utilize simultaneous 2-arm movements (no single-arm dumbbells). Complete full repetitions, 8–10 each; slow concentrated movements; never use more weight than you can handle comfortably.	Take 1–2 multivitamins per day. Include some foods high in fiber to achieve 10–20 grams of fiber intake per day.
BREAST/LYMPH NODE EXCISION	Aerobic modifications remain intact. Exclude pool-related activities until incisions heal sufficiently (3–4 months).	Incorporate flexible tubing and bands for exercising the upper body for at least first 12 weeks. Limit movements to those that utilize both arms simultaneously.	Above recommendations apply.

TREATMENT	AEROBIC ACTIVITY	STRENGTH TRAINING	NUTRITIONAL SUPPORT
BREAST/LYMPH NODE EXCISION CONT'D		Muscle groups to target include forearms, triceps, upper and mid-back muscles. These muscles will specifically support the chest, shoulders, and biceps muscles, which will be most affected by lymph node removal.	

and wives, filled with questions." They were there to demand answers and had a businesslike approach to beating the disease, almost as if they were attending an investment or retirement seminar and looking for the best ways to maximize their dollars or their 401Ks. They understood, as I'm sure you do, too, that information is power—and they wanted plenty of it. More than that, they wanted to take control! It's a far cry from the days when men ignored their health, denied their symptoms, or nodded obediently and did whatever the doctor told them. These men wanted to be involved and active in the management of their disease.

Bob Dole, Michael Milken, Norman Schwarzkopf, Joe Torre, Larry King, Harry Belafonte, Jesse Helms, Hamilton Jordan, Arnold Palmer, Sidney Poitier, Jerry Lewis, Richard Petty . . . the list goes on and on of well-known men diagnosed with prostate cancer, all of them prominent and successful men in their respective fields. These men, and the guys that Jeff met at that meeting, constitute a movement, a movement of men diagnosed with prostate cancer who won't take no for an answer in their efforts to recover.

Although there is nothing yet quite as extensive as a Race for the Cure for prostate cancer, numerous organizations are dedicated to helping men fight back against prostate cancer, including Us Too!, CapCure, Malecare, and the American Cancer Society's Man to Man.

The men behind these organizations, like the ones at that meeting, are inquisitive, motivated, take-charge types. They also tend to be the kind of people who want to charge gung-ho into the FORCE program. Sometimes, we have to pull back on the reins a little bit. Unlike recovery from breast cancer, for which many women are performing exercises within days of their surgery, exercise is not part of the rehab for those who have undergone prostate surgery. In fact, exercise should begin only when the affected area is completely healed and your doctor gives you the green light. Once you can get started, there are also modifications you need to make in our Phase I program:

- Prostate surgery is a major, invasive operation. You want to take plenty of time to allow the healing process to take place and avoid any unnecessary strain on the lower body. So in Phase I, do not do split lunges. When doing chair squats, sit all the way down, instead of just lightly touching the chair.
- In Phase II, after your doctor says it's all right, you can perform the lunges, but without the shopping bags or any extra weight.
- Also in Phase II, skip the modified push-ups, the abdominal crunches, and the double knee stretch hugs.

About twelve weeks after the surgery, you can probably begin to do these exercises, but before you do, ask your doctor. We suggest you add an additional two to three weeks or even a month to Phase I, and incorporate these three very important exercises (push-ups, crunches, and knee hugs) at that point, before moving on to Phase III. See Table 7.2 for more modifications.

The modifications we've discussed for prostate and breast cancer have mostly involved the resistance training exercises. But bicycling is often contraindicated (not recommended) for prostate patients. If you enjoy a leisurely glide around your local park on your bike, fear not, you can probably still do it. In the past, men who had prostate surgery were told by their physicians that biking was completely out of the question. That's not quite true anymore (at least after your initial twelve-week healing period). The traditional bike seat can now be replaced by a new—shall we say, prostate-friendly?—design. It has extra padding and is designed in a way that forces your body forward slightly while you're in the seat, thus taking the strain off the prostate area.

There are several different models and brands for these kinds of seats, ranging from $25 to $100. At this time, we're not aware of studies that have conclusively proved their value; however, we have some anecdotal evidence that these seats work well. If you're interested, it might be worth a trip to the local bike shop, which is where you can buy these seats. If you decide to use one, we suggest riding for just a few minutes your first time out. If you have any signs of discomfort, stop and go back to walking or swimming or any of the other cardiovascular activities you can pursue. If not, then continue—and enjoy one of the best forms of aerobic exercise.

A last word about aerobic exercise and its role in prostate cancer treatment: Although there is no scientific evidence of this, a number of our FORCE program participants were highly fit before being diagnosed with prostate cancer, and, after their surgery and treatment, were able to return quickly to high levels of activity and even competition. According to these FORCE program graduates, the exercise—long-distance running and bicycling sessions of ninety minutes or more—seemed to reduce significantly the side effects of testosterone-blocking drugs. Obviously, if you are not at a high level of physical fitness before your

TABLE 7.2 PROSTATE CANCER REGIMEN

TREATMENT	AEROBIC ACTIVITY	STRENGTH TRAINING	NUTRITIONAL SUPPORT
	(FORCE MODIFICATIONS)	(FORCE MODIFICATIONS)	
PROSTATE CANCER SURGERY AND TREATMENT	Treadmill walking for first 6–8 weeks beginning 6 weeks after surgery, 15–20 min 3 times a week.	2 weeks after surgery, begin upper-body flexibility and stretching exercises, 10–15 min a day (see Chap. 5).	Lower saturated fat to 10% or less. Lower total fat to 20–25% of dietary intake.
	With no treatment, begin walking 4 weeks after surgery for 5–10 min 3 times a week. Treadmill walking 10–15 min a day, first 2 weeks (2–3 times a week).	6 weeks after surgery, begin lower-body flexibility and stretching exercises, 10–15 min a day. Do your stretches in a stationary position lying on the floor or in a chair. With no treatment, begin 4 weeks after surgery.	1 soy product/day (9 grams) for the first 2–4 weeks, 25–35 grams thereafter. Include tofu, soybeans, miso, and soy milk.
	Treadmill walking 20–25 min a day, weeks 2–4 (2–4 times a week).	6 weeks after surgery, begin upper-body weight-bearing exercises, 2 times a week, minimal intensity,	Increase intake of fruits and vegetables. Start with up to 5 servings per day and gradually build up to 9 servings per day.

TREATMENT	AEROBIC ACTIVITY	STRENGTH TRAINING	NUTRITIONAL SUPPORT
PROSTATE CANCER SURGERY AND TREATMENT CONT'D		utilizing 3–7 lbs or following our soup can method (Chap. 5).	
	Treadmill walking 30–40 min a day, weeks 4–8. 15 min warmup, 15 min higher intensity, 10 min cool-down (3–4 times a week).	8 weeks after surgery, begin lower-body weight-bearing exercises, once a week, minimal intensity, utilizing stationary weight equipment or dynabands.	Dietary fiber intake: start slowly with 5–10 grams and gradually increase to 25–35 grams a day.
	Treadmill walking 20–30 min a day, weeks 5–7 (3–4 times a week). Can be substituted with other machines with the exception of a stationary bike, provided you use special seat (see chapter text for more details).	You can maintain this 3 times a week routine, increasing the amount of weight or the number of repetitions. Target large muscle groups, including quadriceps, hamstring, calves, abdominal, chest, deltoid, triceps, and biceps.	Increase weekly intake of tomatoes and tomato-based products. Choose canola and olive oils over other oils.

TREATMENT	AEROBIC ACTIVITY	STRENGTH TRAINING	NUTRITIONAL SUPPORT
PROSTATE CANCER SURGERY AND TREATMENT CONT'D	Treadmill walking 30–40 min a day, weeks 7–10. 15 min warmup, 15 min higher intensity, 10 min cool-down (3–5 times a week).	For the sake of high-endurance workouts, consider high repetitions such as 15–20 and 3–4 sets for each body part.	

surgery, you should not attempt anything more than thirty minutes or so when you start the exercise program. Be gradual and slow in your progression through our posttreatment exercise regimen.

LUNG CANCER

Every year in the United States, more than 164,000 people are diagnosed with lung cancer. Cancers that begin in the lungs are divided into two major types, non-small-cell and small-cell lung cancer, depending on how the cells look under a microscope. Each type of lung cancer spreads in different ways and is treated differently.

Treatment depends on the type of lung cancer, the size, location, and the extent of the tumor, and the general health of the patient. Many different treatments and combinations of treatments may be used to control the cancer and improve the quality of life for the patient. Lung surgery, depending on the factors above, may involve removal of only a small part of the lung, an entire lobe of the lung, or the entire lung. In some cases, the tumor may be inoperable because of the size or location.

The exercise and nutrition modifications we've laid out for you in Table 7.3

TABLE 7.3   LUNG CANCER REGIMEN

TREATMENT	AEROBIC ACTIVITY	STRENGTH TRAINING	NUTRITIONAL SUPPORT
	(FORCE MODIFICATIONS)	(FORCE MODIFICATIONS)	
LUNG SURGERY/TREATMENT	Before surgery: begin walking 5–10 min a day in your home (avoid steps) 5 times a week first 1–4 weeks. After 4–8 weeks, increase to 10–20 min a day. After 8 weeks, continue on treadmill or outside.	Lying flat on your back, apply light pressure to your abdomen with hands. Hands should rise and fall as you exhale through mouth slowly, 10 times a day, 5 times a week, first 2–4 weeks.	During treatment: Eat small, frequent meals every 1–2 hours. Avoid foods low in caloric and protein content (such as soda).
	Seated, slowly raise 1 arm as high as possible, breathing slowly and deliberately, alternate arms, 10 times a day, 5 days a week, 2–4 weeks.	Lying flat with knees bent, exhale completely. Raise each arm individually outward and upward. At top of movement, hold breath 5 seconds. Repeat 5–10 times a day, 5 days per week, for 4–8 weeks.	Maintain or increase fat intake to at least 30% of total dietary intake. Increase protein intake to at least 50% of total dietary intake.
	4 weeks after surgery: In a pool, standing in water at shoulder depth, use overhand	Seated, facing a wall, walk 2 fingers up wall. Walk hand down the wall, breathing slowly	As necessary, include liquid food supplements.

TREATMENT	AEROBIC ACTIVITY	STRENGTH TRAINING	NUTRITIONAL SUPPORT
LUNG SURGERY/TREATMENT CONT'D	swim stroke. Pull back through water with force. Alternate arms, breathe slowly, and repeat 5–10 times a day, 3 times a week.	and alternating arms. Repeat 5 times a day, every day, 2–4 weeks after surgery.	Avoid highly spiced foods and foods high in acidity.
	6–8 weeks after surgery: In a pool, standing in water at shoulder depth, with arms fully extended, palms down, push down through water. Reverse palms and push up through water until surface is broken. Repeat 10 times a day, 3 times a week.	Standing, facing a wall, walk 2 fingers up wall. Walk hand down the wall, breathing slowly and alternating arms. Repeat 5 times a day, every day, 2–4 weeks after surgery.	After treatment: Frequent, small meals with focus on rich nutrients, such as beta carotene, vitamins B, C, E, selenium, and zinc. Decrease saturated fat intake to less than 20% of total fat intake.
	Adhere strictly to breathing recommendations for each movement.	Adhere strictly to breathing recommendations for each movement.	Include 5–9 servings of fruits and vegetables daily. Include protein-rich foods other than red meats.

take into consideration surgery and chemotherapy and call for only breathing exercises in the first two to four weeks or more before surgery.

LEUKEMIA/LYMPHOMA/HODGKIN'S DISEASE

Each year, 30,800 adults and more than 2,600 children in the United States are diagnosed with leukemia; 62,300 are diagnosed under the general heading of lymphoma, including 7,400 with Hodgkin's disease.

Leukemia

is cancer of the blood cells. With this disease, the body produces large numbers of abnormal blood cells, primarily white blood cells. Typically, leukemia is treated with chemotherapy, although some forms do require radiation therapy or bone marrow transplantation.

Lymphoma

is a general term for cancers that develop in the lymphatic system, part of the body's immune system. Lymph is a colorless, watery fluid that contains infection-fighting cells called lymphocytes. The lymphatic system helps the body fight infections and disease. It includes a network of thin tubes that branch into tissues throughout the body. Other portions of this system include lymph nodes, the spleen, thymus, tonsils, and bone marrow.

Hodgkin's disease

is a common type of lymphoma, generally found in people twenty-five years of age and younger. All other lymphomas are grouped together and are known as non-Hodgkin's lymphoma. Lymphomas are treated with chemotherapy, radiation therapy, or bone marrow transplantation, depending on whether the lymphoma is aggressive (high-grade) or indolent (low-grade).

Research has shown that exercise can offset the fatigue caused by the treatment of lymphoma by helping your body produce red blood cells, which can increase oxygen delivery to vital organs. See Table 7.4 for modifications specific to these cancers.

BRAIN TUMORS

Each year, more than 32,000 people in the United States are diagnosed with a brain tumor. The brain is composed of three major parts: the cerebrum, the cerebellum, and the brain stem. Brain tumors can be benign, which means that they do not contain cancer cells but can cause symptoms similar to malignant tumors, which may interfere with vital brain functions and are life-threatening.

Treatment for brain tumors depends on the type, location, and size as well as the patient's age and general health. Brain tumors are treated with surgery, radiation therapy, and chemotherapy. Before treatment occurs, patients may be given steroids to reduce swelling, or anticonvulsant medicine to prevent seizures. Brain surgery is a major operation that may result in general weakness, coordination problems, personality changes, and possible difficulty speaking and thinking.

Patients may require rehabilitation to overcome difficulties in activities of daily living and difficulties with joint weakness. Paralysis and issues with balance may also require physical therapy. This therapeutic approach can last for an extended period of time. We have therefore incorporated exercises in Table 7.5 that are intended to be done while these therapies are progressing.

TABLE 7.4   LEUKEMIA/LYMPHOMA/HODGKIN'S DISEASE REGIMEN

AEROBIC ACTIVITY	STRENGTH TRAINING	NUTRITIONAL SUPPORT
(FORCE MODIFICATIONS)	(FORCE MODIFICATIONS)	
Begin with a 15-min walk 3–4 times a week for 4 weeks. Avoid steps and inclines or walk on a treadmill.	For first 2–4 weeks, 10–15 min of stretching 2–3 times a week.	5–9 servings of fruits and vegetables daily.
Build up to 30 min a day, 4–5 days a week. If possible, alternate days with 30 min on a stationary bicycle.	After 4 weeks of stretching-flexibility movements, begin Phase I weight-bearing exercises (see Chap. 5). Limit weight to 5–10 lbs.	Limit total fat and saturated fat to 20% of total dietary intake.
Gradually increase intensity. Incorporate a 10-min warmup, 15-min increase in intensity, and 10-min cool-down (total 35 min).	After 10 weeks, incorporate Phase II upper and lower body weight-bearing movements with limited intensity and minimal weight.	Include protein-rich foods other than red meat. Total dietary protein intake should equal 40%.
If utilizing heart rate monitor/pulse measurement, maintain effort level of 50–70% of your maximum heart rate.	After 16–18 weeks, gradually increase intensity included in Phase III.	Eat 4–6 smaller meals per day to help your body be more efficient.
Avoid high-impact activities (running, aerobics classes) during treatment. Avoid high-intensity workouts 24 hours before and up to 48 hours after treatments.	Continue to maintain stretching-flexibility movements as you incorporate weight-bearing activities. Reduce intensity 24 hours before and up to 48 hours after treatments.	Maintain a high level of hydration, 8–16 glasses of water per day, especially on exercise days. During treatment and exercising, include sports drinks (Gatorade, All Sport).

TABLE 7.5   BRAIN TUMOR REGIMEN

AEROBIC ACTIVITY	STRENGTH TRAINING	NUTRITIONAL SUPPORT
(FORCE MODIFICATIONS)	(FORCE MODIFICATIONS)	
4 weeks after surgery, begin deep breathing exercises for 4–6 weeks from a seated position (2–4 times a week).	4 weeks after surgery, begin flexibility and stretching exercises, 10–15 min a day (see Chap. 5).	Eat high-caloric meals. If you have a diminished appetite, eat small, frequent meals every 1–2 hours.
After 6 weeks, while seated, breathe in through your nose, raise arms over head slowly, thumbs up. Exhale through your mouth, and slowly lower arms. Repeat 10 times, for 3 sets, 4 days a week.	Lying flat on your back with knees bent, exhale completely. Raise each arm individually outward and upward. At top of movement, hold breath 2–3 seconds. Repeat 5–10 times a day, 3 days a week, 6 weeks after surgery.	Maintain or increase dietary fat to 30% of total dietary intake. During treatment, disregard restrictions on saturated and unsaturated forms of fat.
While seated, place hands on rib cage, push down and in with hands while inhaling deeply through your nose. Breathe out slowly through your mouth. Repeat 10 times, 3 sets, 4 days a week.	Wall volleyball in a chair, preferably with armrests; use inflated balloon and hit against a wall or hit with a friend using your open hand. Play 3 times a week for a few minutes each time (see Chap. 5).	Make your calories count: avoid empty calorie foods like soda, candy, popcorn, and muffins.
Depending on balance issues, use a stationary bicycle, preferably in a recumbent* position, pedal with little or no resistance for 10–15 min 3 times a week for 4–6 weeks.	With a wall, table, or a partner, from a standing position sit down in a chair and stand right back up. Do this slowly, 10 times for 2 sets, 3 days a week, for 3–4 weeks.	Increase protein to at least 50% of total dietary intake. Include protein bars and high-protein drinks to achieve overall increases.

AEROBIC ACTIVITY	STRENGTH TRAINING	NUTRITIONAL SUPPORT
After 6 weeks, increase stationary bicycle riding to 20–30 min including 5 min warmup a cool-down. Increase resistance to raise heart rate to 50–70% of maximum.	Modified push-ups: resting on your knees, push up with your arms 5 times, 2 sets, 3 days a week. Gradually build up to 10 push-ups (see Chap. 5).	During periods of appetite suppression, include liquid food supplements. Include milk and other dairy products as a good source of protein and the best source of calcium.
Include pool exercises such as walking in chest-deep water for 10–15 min and build up to 20–30 min. Use a flotation aid such as an Aquajogger.**	Starting 12 weeks after surgery, follow all Phase I strength training exercises that can be performed in a seated position. After 6 weeks, with doctor's approval, begin Phase I exercises in a standing position.	Avoid foods with high spice content and foods high in acidity. Emphasize foods rich in nutrients such as beta carotene, vitamins B, C, E, selenium, and zinc.

*Recumbent position: reclining position with legs extended with pedals strapped to feet; includes hand rests.
**Aquajogger: a large Styrofoam belt worn around the waist; does not act as a life-preserver but will aid in balance.

IMPORTANT NOTE: As you tire, balance may become an issue. Utilize the help of a partner, personal trainer, or physical therapist. Begin slowly and gradually, and be patient.

After side effects from surgery lessen, gradually incorporate dietary recommendations in Chapter 6.

COLORECTAL CANCER

Together, cancers of the colon and rectum, also called colorectal cancer, are among the most common cancers in the United States, affecting 130,200 men and women each year. It is most commonly diagnosed among people who are over the age of fifty. The colon and rectum are parts of the body's digestive system, which removes nutrients from food and stores waste until it passes out of the body. The colon makes up the first six feet of the large intestine, and the rectum is located in the last eight to ten inches. Treatment depends mainly on the size, location, and extent of the tumor.

Several different methods are often used in combination to treat colorectal disease. These include surgery, chemotherapy, radiation therapy, and biological therapies.

Our exercise program, shown in Table 7.6, takes into consideration surgical interventions and the ensuing side effects along with other localized and systemic forms of treatment.

TABLE 7.6 COLORECTAL CANCER REGIMEN

AEROBIC ACTIVITY	STRENGTH TRAINING	NUTRITIONAL SUPPORT
(FORCE MODIFICATIONS)	(FORCE MODIFICATIONS)	
Begin walking 5–10 min a day in your home 2 weeks after surgery 4 times a week (avoid steps). After 4–6 weeks, increase to 10–20 min a day 4–5 times a week.	4 weeks after surgery, incorporate upper-body flexibility and stretching exercises, 10–15 min a day, 2–3 times a week (see Chap. 5).	Lower saturated fat to 10% or less. Lower total fat to 20–25% of dietary intake.
After 6 weeks, walk either on a treadmill or outside for 15–30 min a day, 3–4 days a week.	8 weeks after surgery, begin lower-body flexibility and stretching exercises, 10–15 min a day. Stretch this muscle group only in a stationary position, such as lying on the floor or in a chair.	1 soy product per day (9 grams) for the first 2–4 weeks, 25–35 grams thereafter. Include servings of soy milk, tofu, and miso in place of animal foods.
After 12 weeks, walk outside for 30–40 min a day, 3–4 times a week. Include a 10-min warmup and 5–10 min cool-down.	6 weeks after surgery, begin upper-body weight-bearing exercises, 2 times a week, minimal intensity, utilizing no more than 3–7 lbs or following our soup can method (see Chap. 5).	Increase intake of fruits and vegetables. Start with up to 5 servings a day and gradually build up to 5–9 servings a day. Include cruciferous vegetables like broccoli, cabbage, and cauliflower.

AEROBIC ACTIVITY	STRENGTH TRAINING	NUTRITIONAL SUPPORT
After 12 weeks, you may also supplement with water aerobics that utilize upper and lower body muscles 2 days a week. Or walk in chest-deep water for 15 min.	8–10 weeks after surgery, begin lower-body weight-bearing exercises, 1 time a week, minimal intensity, 8–10 repetitions, utilizing stationary weight equipment or flexible tubing or bands. You can maintain this 2–3 times a week routine, increasing the amount of weight or the number of repetitions.	Dietary fiber intake: start slowly with 5–10 grams and gradually increase to 25–35 grams per day. Include fish high in omega-6 fatty acid contained in salmon, tuna, mackerel, and sardines. Include folate each day, found in orange juice, lentils, asparagus, and a multivitamin containing folic acid. Include vitamin D, which has been linked to lower colon cancer rates.

CHAPTER EIGHT

THE K-FORCE PROGRAM FOR CHILDREN

This year, about 13,000 children and teenagers will be diagnosed with cancer. When you as a parent first hear the word "leukemia" or "brain tumor," life is changed forever. Bear in mind, however, that cancers affecting children and adolescents are quite different from the malignant diseases affecting adults.

The good news is that at least 75 percent of these young people can be treated effectively and *cured*.

The idea of developing a version of the FORCE program for kids was inspired by Jeff Blatnick, the 1984 Olympic gold medal–winning wrestler. If Blatnick performed in a higher-profile sport, there would probably be books and a movie based on his life, so inspiring is his example. Two years before the Olympics, he was diagnosed with Hodgkin's disease. After a series of daily radiation treatments, he resumed his rigorous training. In one of the most memorable images of the 1984 Games, Blatnick dropped to his knees on the mat and put his hands together in thanks after winning the match that gave him the gold. So moving was Blatnick's achievement, his teammates elected him to carry the U.S. flag in the closing ceremonies.

But that wasn't the end of the story. A year later, Blatnick was again diagnosed with Hodgkin's. He went through six months of chemotherapy—showing up for his last injection on Valentine's Day 1986 wearing a tuxedo—and has been cancer-free ever since.

Early in 1995, Jeff Berman asked Blatnick to speak to his Athletes Support Group for Cancer, the forerunner of the FORCE program. "He said, 'You know, Jeff, I can certainly help adults, but if you had kids, I'd much rather work with them,' " recalls Berman.

At that point, the only people involved in the program were adults. But at about the same time he had this discussion with the former Olympic wrestler, Berman paid a visit to Memorial Sloan-Kettering Cancer Center in Manhattan and noticed some of the kids there. He put two and two together. "I realized that I couldn't change their lives, couldn't fix their cancer, but I could at least give them one day when they'd feel better, forget about their disease and their treatment."

So he organized the first Kids Sports Day. On a beautiful spring afternoon in 1995, about sixty kids from the Ronald McDonald House in Manhattan, all of them with cancer, spent an afternoon with some special people. They rode bikes with Nancy Powers, an Olympic-caliber cyclist who has a brain tumor, and ran up and down 73rd Street (which had been closed off for the day) with Mark Conover, the 1988 Olympic marathoner who has Hodgkin's disease. Most memorably of all, they grappled with Blatnick, who spread out a mat, got on his knees, and wrestled about a dozen kids at a time. Big, small, timid, bold, they came flying at him, and with the grace of the champion—not to mention a touch of the showman—he gently "pinned" them all (of course, with much tickling and laughing).

One message from all this: Even big, strong guys can get cancer—and they can still be big and strong and win gold medals afterward. Another, more immediate message: This kind of active play, wrestling, is fun (and, unlike the garish, professional version that's so popular these days, it's real).

Sports Day is now an annual event, attracting hundreds of children. And

Blatnick's en masse wrestling match is still one of the highlights. But watching the first one in 1995, seeing the kids running around, wrestling, biking, laughing—basically, being kids—Berman learned an important lesson. "I realized that these kids want to play, want to keep doing what they've been doing, despite their cancer," he said. "People view that as being brave, sort of laughing in the face of catastrophe. But the kids don't. They view it as being normal."

It's normal for all children to want to get out and move and be active. This is also one of the core principles of the FORCE program for adults. Berman believed that the same foundation—stress or anxiety management, proper nutrition, and physical activity—could help children as well. When he began discussing it with experts in the field, the answer came back a resounding yes. Most enthusiastic of all was Genevieve Lowry, a certified child life specialist at New York Presbyterian Hospital, who became the coordinator of the new K-FORCE program for kids six to twelve years of age, which was launched in spring 2000.

We're often asked the philosophy of the K-FORCE program, but we couldn't possibly articulate it any better than Lowry did, in remarks she made at a fundraising reception at New York's Four Seasons hotel in early 2000. Here's what she said:

> When I tell people that I work with kids and cancer, I always get the same response. "Isn't that depressing?" And I always give the same answer. "No, it's not."
>
> There is nothing sad and depressing about children's laughter in the face of hardship because they don't know it's hard. There is nothing more inspiring than a child who knows what is really important in life . . . Pokémon.
>
> And there is nothing that says "I am brave" better than a Band-Aid.
>
> K-FORCE will give back to children some of the things they lose during a life-threatening illness, such as a sense of belonging, control, and self-esteem. The combined components of exercise, nutrition, and relaxation,

plus the children's inherent strengths—their resiliency, their unique and often uncomplicated look at life—work together to help them recover the essence of childhood.

Look at it this way: What kid doesn't like to be part of something fun, something that involves a lot of playing and running around, a lot of imagination and creativity, not to mention eating some ice cream once in a while? That's what the K-FORCE program is all about: teaching children valuable coping skills, helping them feel better through activity and proper eating, while remembering that they are still kids.

And that's what we must remember: they *are* kids. Not sick kids, but kids. It's we, the adults, who in our caring, well-meaning way apply that label (they're "sick") and show it in our words and actions. The children themselves see it differently: they're able to put their disease aside and still return to the most important business at hand—being kids.

We try to reflect that difference in the K-FORCE program. Which is why it's much more group-oriented (because kids love to play with other kids) and much less structured (because kids are not likely to count fat grams or calculate their maximum heart rate). One other important difference is that *you*, the parent, are involved. In the adult FORCE program, participants seek the consent and support of their loved ones as they make changes in their diet and activity patterns, but they don't need anyone else's consent. Kids in the FORCE program can't get along without your consent, though. They require that guiding hand.

Of course, we know you can't entirely replicate the environment or all the recommendations of our eight-week K-FORCE program at home. But you can apply some of the same principles and use some of the activities and games that our K-FORCE professionals use in your own home. And you can learn, as we have, not to dwell on the child's sickness, but to encourage his or her wellness. You can learn, as we have, not to bemoan the illness of a child, but instead to concentrate our energies on allowing that child to experience and celebrate childhood—and that means learning, playing, having fun.

PHASE I: RELAXATION AND EXPRESSIVE ARTS

The purpose of this phase of the program, the kids' counterpart to adult stress management, is to help them use their inherent creativity to develop visualization and imagery skills. These, in turn, can help reduce anxiety and anxiousness associated with their treatments. Psychologists do this with adults all the time (and we do something similar in the adult relaxation drills in the FORCE program), but kids aren't necessarily going to be able to close their eyes, clear their minds, and imagine waves gently lapping a tropical beach. We need to fire up their imaginations—and we do that through a couple of fun activities you can do at home.

THE IMAGINATION SCRAPBOOK

This exercise starts with a blank page in a scrapbook or notebook. On top of the first page, ask your child to think of a place, real or imagined, that he or she would like to visit or has visited. Then have the child write down the name of this wonderful place (you can help with the spelling!). On page 2, ask the child to draw a picture of what it looks like. Page 3: What are the smells and sounds you'd hear there? Page 4: Write or draw some of the things you'd eat while you're there. Page 5: What does it feel like? Finally, on the last page, ask your child to think of a time when he or she might want to visit this place—in his or her mind.

Depending on the age of your child, this process could take a few minutes more or less per page. That's okay. The speed of the child's response isn't what's important. The purpose is to help him or her sharpen the skill of visualization. The more senses you involve, the more vivid and real the imagery becomes. So that the next time your son or daughter faces an anxious moment—say, a procedure or a hospital visit—you can encourage him or her to visit the places written about in the imagination scrapbook.

By the way, you might get something out of this, too. For example, Genevieve learned, from one of her ten-year-old students, that the moon smells like gingerbread and marshmallows. How come Neil Armstrong didn't notice that?

SHAKE YOUR STRESS AWAY

Progressive muscle relaxation is a technique commonly used in stress management programs, including the adult FORCE program (see Chapter 4). But kids aren't likely to have the patience to approach this in the more logical, deliberate way we do as grown-ups. "Kids are much more physical," says Genevieve. "Taking deep breaths and imagining your stress away doesn't make much sense to them."

Instead, you want to be "loose like a wet noodle." To get rid of the stress, Genevieve has her kids jump up and down, wiggle their legs, and shake the stress off their bodies, like puppy dogs throwing water off themselves after a bath. Shake your arms, your legs. Help them make the connection by telling them, "The things you're worrying about, you're shaking off you!" (And of course, you should be doing this right along with your kids!)

Just a few minutes are all you need for this. And remember: The goal here is to teach them a skill. Any time they're nervous, they can "shake their stress away."

HAPPY NEW YEAR!

Deep breathing is a quick, easy way to manage your own stress, as we learned in Chapter 4. But, Lowry notes, inhaling and exhaling deeply has been shown to help dissipate acute pain—for example, the pain of an injection. Again, kids aren't likely to sit still for the kind of deep breathing drills we recommend for adults. So try this: Get one of those "party blowers." You know, the New Year's Eve party favors that, when you blow into them, unfold and make a funny noise (or get a pinwheel or any other fun little toy that forces children to take deep breaths and expel). Encourage them to do this a few times, again at home, in a relaxed setting (and if you want to yell "Happy New Year!" even if it's the middle of May, fine. That's part of the fun). This will help show them the value of deep breathing any time of the year.

When they need to take a deep breath—again, perhaps, before getting a shot—ask them to pretend that it's December 31 all over again. Before they can say "Happy New Year," the breath is drawn and expelled and the shot's been delivered.

ADDITIONAL TIPS FOR PARENTS

Here are a few other tips for parents, to help manage your child's anxiety:

• When kids need to be brave, you can tell them that a battery gets charged up, just the way courage does: from energy they can get by simply holding hands or hugging their parents. Explains Genevieve: "This contact helps children who have a hard time sitting still. A parent who hugs the child and says 'I'm giving you my bravery and courage,' is actually helping to calm him or her down without the child feeling as if he or she is being restrained."

• In general, Lowry recommends that children fighting cancer should be treated as normally as possible. "When you whisper in front of the child or don't behave as you used to, that sends a message," she says. "And the message is that something is really wrong, because Mommy and Daddy aren't treating me as they did before." Normal treatment should include rewards and even punishment, if warranted: "If you punished them before for misbehavior, they should not think they can act out without consequences. Don't spoil them, because they'll survive and you'll end up with spoiled brats."

• Maintain a regular schedule: Give children their medication or dressing changes the same time every day. If the children can't go to school, get them up and dressed as if they could. "Keeping a daily routine is how kids hold on to normalcy," says Lowry.

PHASE II: PHYSICAL ACTIVITY

Physical activity—simply getting out and moving—should be a part of every child's life, whether or not he or she has cancer.

Back in the days before we worried about high cholesterol, resting heart rates, and children's obesity, we had another term for children's physical activity. It was called "play." Active play. "That's what we did when I was growing up," says John Buzzerio, exercise physiologist for the FORCE program. "My dad used to give us a can and we'd kick the can around. We'd go out and play hide-and-seek. Simple stuff."

That simple, back-to-basics stuff, Buzzerio believes, should form the basis of an activity program for every child. But you need to take some precautions. First, you'll need to get permission from your physician. You may have to monitor blood counts, make sure that the child—especially a child going through chemotherapy—drinks plenty of water before, during, and after exercise. If the child has physical limitations, you'll obviously need to work around those as you help plan those activities. But—as thousands of physically challenged men and women, boys and girls who are actively pursuing competitive sports remind us every day—being on crutches or in a wheelchair is no reason not to get out and be active.

Time is a relative thing in kids' exercise. Although experts recommend sixty minutes a day of activity for children, they don't mean sixty minutes nonstop on a treadmill. A few minutes here, a few minutes there can be just as effective—and is probably a more natural activity pattern—for children. What's more important is that you monitor them closely. During our K-FORCE sessions, trainer Regina Grieco constantly asks the children, "Are you tired?" Similarly, you should make sure to monitor your child's level of fatigue.

Getting up and moving—as far as they can, as often as they can—is as therapeutic for children with cancer as it is for adults. It's just got to be a lot simpler and a lot less structured. Here are some ways to encourage it for children on a daily basis.

HAVE YOU PLAYED TODAY?

It doesn't have to be competitive. It doesn't have to involve teams or technology or even bats, balls, and coaches. Simply playing active games, as John used to when he played kick-the-can as a kid, counts as activity. And in some cases, for example, compared to a competitive youth baseball game where the talented kids play and the others sit on the bench, playing a game of tag or hide-and-seek in the backyard might actually be *more* vigorous and beneficial, because everybody gets to participate. If your child has siblings or friends the same age in the neighborhood, encourage them all to play together. If not, well . . . when's the last time you had a rousing game of hide-and-seek?

SET AN ACTIVE EXAMPLE

Children learn by example. If Mom or Dad spends precious free time on the couch, then it takes no great intellect to predict where their children will probably end up. On the other hand, if they see you heading out the door in the morning for a run, a walk, or a trip to the gym, they'll be influenced in a more positive and active way.

Perhaps the best way to nudge your child down the road toward an active lifestyle is to set out on that road together. Make some of the time you spend with your child *active* time. Ride your bikes together around the neighborhood; take a hike together in your local park. Buzzerio recalls that when his daughter Kristy (now fourteen) was a child, Saturday morning was "their" time, and they'd use that time to take walks together. "She was about four years old," recalls Buzzerio. "In the middle of the walk, I'd say 'Come on, Kristy, let's run a little.' We would run for a minute or so, and then I'd stop and act as if I were out of breath. Then when she stopped, I'd suddenly start running again. She'd giggle and chase me, and then she'd do the same thing to me. If we were adults, we would have called this 'speed training' or 'interval work.' But with her, it was just fun, it was playing, and she didn't even realize she was exercising."

LET'S GET SILLY!

If you're forced to stay indoors, no problem. Just think "aerobic dancing" without the aerobic part. In other words, just put on a tape or crank up the music, and shake your booty. Kids love to dance—the sillier the better. And although no one's counting repetitions or rate of perceived exertion, it's still movement, it's fun, and it's time spent together. That's good medicine for your kids . . . and for you.

PUSH UP, STEP UP FOR IMPROVED STRENGTH

Strength training, as we learned in Chapter 5, doesn't have to involve free weights or machines. Body-weight exercises are a great way for kids to begin to increase their strength and fitness. Buzzerio recommends two basic exercises for K-FORCE home participants: push-ups (modified, if necessary; see Chapter 5 for a description of these) and step-ups.

Basically, step-ups are a version of the Step or bench aerobics classes that are so popular in health clubs. For your child, though, the aim is not a forty-five-minute, cardiovascular workout, but a basic strengthening exercise for the lower body. It's simple, and, always a factor when dealing with children, it's fun. Standing in front of a staircase in your house, step up the height of one step, or about six inches, with the left leg, then with the right. (Don't overstep: You don't want the knee to extend beyond the toes, as this will put undue stress on the knee.) Then step down with the left and down with the right. Buzzerio suggests that you do this exercise—repeating the steps in an up-up-down-down sequence—to music. Keep it to a few minutes, at least in the beginning. And, as with any other exercise, let your child tell you when he or she is fatigued. "No pain, no gain" is no way to train kids.

PHASE III: NUTRITION

Let's face it: kids aren't really interested in nutrition. They want foods that taste great and are fun to eat. And yet, we know that a healthy diet—one that is low in fat, high in fiber, and rich in fruits and vegetables—is as important to kids as it is to adults. Eating a healthier diet will help children in the battle against cancer, just as it helps adults. And there's this benefit, too: when they go into remission, they will already have the foundation of a good diet that will help protect them in the future.

Parents face a frustrating task in getting kids to eat right, because it's difficult to know what they're eating when they're at school or at a friend's home. The secret? "Fill your home with a variety of delicious and healthy choices, and encourage children to make their own decisions from among these foods," suggests FORCE nutritionist Heather Salomon. "Once they begin to enjoy the choices provided at home, there's a much better chance they'll make more of these choices when they're outside the home." Also, Heather suggests, get the children involved in the process. Bring them with you shopping and teach them to read labels; explain why you're choosing certain foods in the supermarket.

Some of the foods you should keep in the house are fresh fruits, low-fat yogurt and low-fat cheeses, raw vegetable sticks, crunchy whole wheat crackers, fun-shaped graham crackers, pretzels, and cereals. Use them for snacks and for meals. We've included many low-fat, high-fiber foods in the suggestions in Table 8.1. However, while we stress this as part of a healthy diet for kids (and adults, as you saw in Chapter 6), keep in mind that in some cases—particularly if your child is experiencing side effects from treatment or is underweight—the emphasis should be on foods your child can tolerate, regardless of whether the foods are lower in fat or not. If you have doubts about what to feed your child, make sure you consult with your physician.

TABLE 8.1   K-FORCE NUTRITION

Breakfast

Your child no doubt has a favorite breakfast cereal. (What kid doesn't, given the bombardment of TV commercials for these products?) Fine, don't fight it. Work with it.

Try to mix a higher-fiber cereal or granola with his or her favorite, or add some berries or bananas.

Mix child's favorite granola or fruit or add raisins into yogurt.

Mix child's favorite chopped vegetables into eggs and omelets.

Keep whole wheat or seven-grain bread in the house, instead of just white bread.

Lunch/Dinner

Make sandwiches or wraps from low-fat ingredients (e.g., turkey breast or grilled chicken).

Prepare tuna salad with low-fat mayo or add celery for an added "crunch."

Make your own pizzas and top them with a variety of vegetables and plenty of tomato sauce but low-fat cheese.

Make your own tacos with soft flour tortillas and add salsa, turkey or chicken meat, beans, onions, peppers, tomatoes, dark lettuce, and low-fat cheeses. Let your kids make their own!

Add spices, lemon, or low-fat sauces to vegetables for more flavor.

Replace ground meat in recipes with ground turkey breast (e.g., in chili, casseroles, meat loaf).

Prepare pasta dishes and mix vegetables into the tomato-based marinara sauce.

Add chopped vegetables to macaroni and cheese.

Snacks

Stock up on the sensible choices, such as:

Frozen bananas/grapes
Fresh fruits
Raisins
Pretzels
Flavored rice cakes
Whole wheat crackers with low-fat cheese
Low-fat yogurts
Low-fat granola
Fig bars
Graham crackers
Raw vegetables dipped in low-fat dressing or dip made with low-fat/fat-free sour cream
Air-popped or low-fat flavored popcorn
Frozen fruit bar

And try these simple snack recipes:

TRAIL MIX: Add pretzels, cereal, and raisins in a bowl and toss together.
FRUIT SMOOTHIE: Blend ½ cup skim milk, 2 ice cubes, and pieces of fresh fruit (e.g., peaches, mangos, pineapple) until mixed evenly.
PUDDING KISSES: Drop spoonfuls of chocolate pudding (made with nonfat milk) onto wax paper: Freeze and enjoy!
CINNAMON APPLE WEDGES: Cut 1 small apple into wedges, sprinkle with a mixture of cinnamon and ½ tsp sugar.
YOGURT POP: Punch a wooden stick through a 6-oz cup of nonfat/low-fat fruit yogurt and freeze.
FRUITY POPCORN: Use 1 cup of air-popped popcorn and 1 Tbsp dried mixed fruit or raisins. Mix well and serve.

LISTEN TO YOUR CHILD

Athletes talk about "listening" to their bodies, in other words, monitoring them-selves and being alert to signs of fatigue or injury. Their bodies will "tell" them when to stop and when to go harder. Similarly, pediatric nutrition specialists Elena Ladas, MS, and Deborah Kennedy, MS, remind us that one of the most dif-ficult changes parents encounter in a child with cancer is therapy-induced changes in appetite. "It's important to realize that children's appetites will go through stages," says Ladas. "There will be times when they're too sick to eat. Other times, alterations in their sense of taste and smell will make them dislike foods they once enjoyed. Conversely, there may be periods when your child is ravenous, eating you out of house and home!"

To deal with this, Ladas stresses the importance of *listening to your child*. Specifically: Don't force food if he or she is not hungry. Rather, make each meal count:

- Top toast with butter, peanut butter, or both.
- Sprinkle wheat germ over cereal or in soup.
- Take advantage of the times when your child is feeling well: Cook nutrient-dense, healthy, whole foods.

It's also important to work with a nutritionist during these phases in order to develop a plan that is modified to your child's specific needs. A nutritionist should be part of your child's cancer care management team. If you do not cur-rently have one, contact your physician or your hospital. Another good source for general information on nutrition or to find a qualified dietitian in your area is the American Dietetic Association. Call their Consumer Nutrition Hot Line at 800-366-1655 or visit their Web site at *www.eatright.org*.

ON THE ROAD TO A
HEALTHY FUTURE . . . TOGETHER

We've detailed many of the things you can do to help increase children's activity level, improve diet, and manage anxiety levels. But, as they go through treatment, there are other things you need to do—for their health and yours, for now, and for the times ahead.

DO UNTO YOUR CHILDREN
AS YOU DO UNTO YOURSELF

The importance of setting an example for your children cannot be overstated. Here's an interesting observation: Researchers some years ago found that the strongest predictor of whether a child will become a dedicated reader was not books in the home, the influence of a teacher, trips to the public library, or reading aloud at bedtime. It was the presence of a daily newspaper in the house. A child observes a parent reading for knowledge, information, and entertainment. This is done without any fanfare during the course of the day. The information is often practical. Immersed in this environment, the child will want to emulate Mom and Dad and the need to read on a daily basis. This way of learning applies equally to diet, exercise, sleep habits, and other healthy lifestyle choices.

Children inherently want to move, to play, to socialize, to explore, to show affection. There are a lot of reasons to work as a family to reinforce these behaviors and promote healthy lifestyle choices. One of the most important is the fact that there are medical conditions (including second cancers, heart problems, and metabolic disorders) that can develop years (if not decades) after treatment for childhood cancer. For example, teenage girls are treated and cured of Hodgkin's disease or non-Hodgkin's lymphoma with radiotherapy aimed at lymph nodes within the chest. These girls have a markedly increased risk (thirty-eight times greater than the population at large) for the future development of breast cancer, due to the carcinogenic potential of radiation to the developing breast tissue. Exercise and dietary measures may potentially reduce the risk.

As the ranks of childhood cancer survivors march into adulthood, we want to do everything possible to help them achieve excellent health. It therefore makes a lot of sense to think preventively and—as a family unit—make healthy lifestyle decisions. A varied diet rich in fruits and vegetables and low in fat may help prevent cancer from striking again. Regular exercise also reduces the risk. And avoiding carcinogens—tobacco, excess sunlight, and excess alcohol—makes good sense for the entire family unit.

AIM HIGH AND FOCUS ON YOUR GOALS

It is important to look ahead and imagine that the end of the treatment phase is the beginning of the rest of your child's life. And it is important to strive for the highest possible performance goals, expecting the best from your cancer care specialists and also from your child. We are often amazed by the progress kids can make in physical therapy and in their academic performance when they are encouraged and expected to meet high standards. Don't hold back: Focus on the long-term goals and work hard to achieve them. Encourage your child to join a soccer team, a support group, and summer camp programs. Seek out the most talented and dedicated specialists, whether it's your doctor, your college counselor, or your social worker. Help your child go for the gold!

PRESERVE THE UNIQUENESS

Having successfully navigated the cancer experience, most parents and patients want to put the whole thing behind them. To some extent, this is feasible. But now is the time to be certain to gather the details of the diagnostic testing and treatment in a file that can be maintained and updated. Unlike other, more commonplace childhood conditions, such as chicken pox or strep throat, there will be lifelong reminders of the oncology experience and a need to keep a medical file. It's like the need to have a record of childhood immunizations.

Most children are far too young to comprehend their illness or the specifics of treatment. Many intricate details of the treatment, including the names of specific medications and their doses, are easily forgotten or never obtained by the family. When we are alive and healthy, basking in the sheer exhilaration of it all, it's easy to deny ever having had a serious, often life-threatening illness.

But for your child, this information is critically important, and it's therefore up to you to preserve the uniqueness of the treatment experience. Create a scrapbook, a file, a disc with all of the "vital statistics." Be sure to maintain regular contact with a team of experts who understand the ongoing needs of childhood cancer survivors.

Most of all, continue to give your child the most important things of all: your love and support.

AFTERWORD

Jeff Berman, Force Program Founder

While this book was in its final stages of completion, I went through a four-month cycle of chemotherapy.

Going into this round of chemotherapy—my third since I was diagnosed in 1990, and my first since 1997—I went back to my personal basics: a nutrition refresher course with Heather Salomon, several visits to my social work friends at the Post-Treatment Resource Program at Memorial Sloan-Kettering Cancer Center, sessions with my own psychologist, and discussions with FORCE exercise physiologist John Buzzerio to modify my exercise regime. In other words, I went through everything that we recommended for you in this book.

I'd be less than honest if I told you it was a breeze. Part of my protocol involved a new form of treatment known as a monoclonal antibody, and I went through a few difficult days. But the bottom line is that I was better prepared to deal with this through my good physical conditioning. I was better able to handle the effects of the drugs and the stress of the treatment because of my diet and my ability to utilize some of those same relaxation drills we recommend in Chapter 4.

Now, three weeks after the last treatment, I'm feeling good, I'm eating well, I'm back to work. So, once again, I'm living proof that the FORCE program works!

How did I cope during some of the dark periods? I tried to maintain a balance between eating well when I could and slacking off when I had to. I built my exercise regimen around my weekly chemotherapy schedule. I modified the intensity and duration of the exercise, and took days off when I was really wiped out.

I learned—or perhaps relearned—some things that may help you in the future. For one, I was reminded of the body's resilience, especially the resilience of the body that's as strong as it can be, the body that has been well cared for. That, of course, is one of the essential lessons of the FORCE program: We can better deal with our treatment when we're in better physical condition.

But there are other aspects of this disease and how to deal with it that I had time to think about. When people make generous offers, such as prayers, hospital visits, and get-well wishes, accept it, allow them to be generous. When you receive an offer of assistance at home or work, with the kids or errands around town, say yes. Your acceptance of such offers and well-meaning assistance does not constitute a failure on your part. If anything, you'll benefit both physically and psychologically by the relief it will give you.

Last, I'm convinced that the way to get through chemo with your health and sanity intact is to keep a balanced perspective. If you have a good day, don't overdo it, because that can lead to several bad days. If you're not feeling well, remember that tomorrow's another day. Don't allow any medical professionals to dismiss your physical and psychological ailments. They're real to you—and if you speak up, you might find that there is a way to address these issues.

The FORCE program is about taking action and doing things to help yourself. But during my recent treatment, I was reminded that there are times when inaction or avoidance is a better strategy. For example, don't answer your phone if you don't feel up to it. Ask the people close to you for some space or privacy if you need it. Politely hold off any visitors if you don't want them.

But above all, you've got to stick with it. I did, and now I'm starting to feel like my old self. That's the secret—in treatment, and in the FORCE program. So now, it's your turn to see if these principles will work for you. You have to take the proverbial bull by the horns and make some changes in your diet, your activity, the way you approach each day. You can't look back; you can't alter what has already happened. But you can take the set of plans we've provided you and use them to reconstruct your life.

Are you ready to do that? Do you want to take some control over the management of your disease? Do you want to fight back? Do you want to make yourself stronger and healthier even as your body fights this disease? You can! We're confident that you will, and that, a few months from now, you'll be writing to tell us about your success story in the FORCE program.

On behalf of my friend and favorite writer John Hanc and coauthor Dr. Fran Fleegler and the entire FORCE advisory board, I wish you good luck!

RESOURCES

NEW YORK METRO AREA

Achilles Track Club
42 West 38th Street, 4th Fl.
New York, NY 10018
212-354-0300
www.achillestrackclub.org
International organization dedicated to helping people with any type of disability get involved with running and physical activity.

Adelphi University New York Statewide Breast Cancer Support Hotline
Adelphi University School of Social Work
Garden City, NY 11530
800-877-8077
516-877-4444
www.adelphi.edu/nysbchot
Goals are to educate, support, empower, and advocate for breast cancer patients, professionals, and the community.

Cancer Care, Inc.
275 Seventh Avenue
New York, NY 10001
212-221-3300 or 212-302-2400
800-813-HOPE (4673)
www.cancercare.org
Support, outreach, education, and referrals for people and families living with cancer.

Cancer Support Services, Inc.
216 East 77th Street, 5C
New York, NY 10021
212-628-9728
www.cancersupport.org
Organization of FORCE Program founder, Jeff Berman.

Creative Center for Women with Cancer, Inc.
147 West 26th Street, 6th floor
New York, NY 10001
646-336-7612
www.ccwconline.org

Friends in Deed
594 Broadway, Suite 706
New York, NY 10012
212-925-2009
www.friendsindeed.org
Provides support for anyone with a life-threatening illness and their families, friends, and caregivers; anyone dealing with grief and loss; and all those facing critical life challenges.

Friends of Karen
800-637-2774
New York–based organization serving the NYC Metro area that offers support for families and children facing cancer.

Holistic Approaches to Cancer Care
1047 Amsterdam Avenue
New York, NY 10025
212-316-7436
Workshops offering free, high-quality educational programs on holistic therapies and
their uses in cancer care.

Post Treatment Resource Program
Memorial Sloan-Kettering Cancer Center
215 East 68th Street, Ground Floor
New York, NY 10021
212-717-3527
www.mskcc.org
Free service offering a variety of community-based educational workshops and lectures
and support programs for cancer patients and their families.

Project S.H.E. (BWBCAF)
467 West 143rd Street, Suite 3
New York, NY 10031
www.projectshe.org
The purpose of this organization is to bring awareness to the African-American community about breast cancer.

SHARE
1501 Broadway, Suite 1720
New York, NY 10036
212-719-0364
www.sharecancersupport.org
Self-help for women with breast and ovarian cancer. Provides emotional and social support services to women with breast or ovarian cancer and their families and friends.

The Valerie Fund
2101 Millburn Avenue
Maplewood, NJ 07040
973-761-0422
www.thevaleriefund.org
The Valerie Fund's mission is to help provide financial support for the comprehensive medical care of children with cancer and blood disorders.

With You In Mind
314 Wadsworth Avenue
New York, NY 10040-0420
212-568-7165
An organization dedicated to post-mastectomy support group services.

Young Survival Coalition
Box 528, 52 A Carmine Street
New York, NY 10014
800-972-1011
212-916-7667
www.youngsurvival.org
The only international network of breast cancer survivors and supporters dedicated to the critical concerns and issues unique to young women with breast cancer.

NATIONAL/INTERNATIONAL

Alliance for Lung Cancer Advocacy, Support, and Education (ALCASE)
P.O. Box 849
Vancouver, WA 98666
800-298-2436
www.alcase.org
ALCASE is the only nonprofit organization dedicated solely to helping people living with lung cancer improve the quality of their lives through advocacy, support, and education.

American Cancer Society

800-ACS-2345

www.cancer.org

Programs include:

Man-to-Man-Outreach, education and support for men with prostate cancer; and Sister-to-Sister-Outreach, education and support for African-American women with breast cancer.

CAnCare of Houston

9575 Katy Freeway, Suite 428

Houston, TX 77024

713-461-0028

www.cancare.org

CAnCare is comprised of people with cancer experiences who are trained and assigned to give quality time to a cancer patient or family member.

Cancer Kids

P.O. Box 2715

Waxahachie, TX 75168

www.cancerkids.org

Helping children with cancer tell their stories to the world.

Candlelighters Childhood Cancer Foundation

3910 Warner Street

Kensington, MD 20895

800-366-2223

www.candlelighters.org

Dedicated to parents of children who are being treated for or have been affected by cancer.

Casting For Recovery
PMB N257
946 Great Plain Avenue
Needham, MA 02492-3030
888-553-3500
www.castingforrecovery.org
Fly-fishing retreats for women recovering from breast cancer.

Cure for Lymphoma Foundation
215 Lexington Avenue
New York, NY 10016
800-CFL-6848
212-213-9595
www.cfl.org
A nationwide nonprofit organization dedicated to funding research and providing support and education for those whose lives have been touched by Hodgkin's disease.

Gilda's Club Worldwide
322 Eighth Avenue, Suite 1402
New York, NY 10001
212-686-9898
www.gildasclub.org
Gilda's Club offers support and networking groups, lectures, workshops, and social events in a nonresidential, homelike setting free of charge to people with cancer and their families.

Lance Armstrong Foundation
P.O. Box 13026
Austin, TX 78711
512-236-8820
www.laf.org
The foundation provides information, services, and support to help cancer patients manage and survive cancer.

Leukemia and Lymphoma Society

1311 Mamaroneck Avenue

White Plains, NY 10605

914-949-5213

800-955-4572

www.leukemia-lymphoma.org

The society is committed to providing information, support, and guidance to persons living with blood-related cancers and to health professionals involved in their care.

Medical Health and Fitness

P.O. Box 29

Santa Barbara, CA 93102

888-880-5227

www.medhealthfit.com

Dedicated to improving the health of people with chronic diseases through educational materials and product lines.

NABCO (National Alliance of Breast Cancer Organizations)

9 East 37th Street, 10th Floor

New York, NY 10016

888-806-2226

www.nabco.org

A nonprofit resource for information about breast cancer, providing current research, treatment options, support referrals, and links.

National Children's Cancer Society

1015 Locust, Suite 600

St. Louis, MO 63101

800-532-6459

www.children-cancer.com

It's mission is to improve the quality of life for children with cancer and to reduce the risk of cancer through financial and in-kind assistance, advocacy, support services, and education.

The Susan G. Komen Breast Cancer Foundation
5005 LBJ Freeway, Suite 250
Dallas, TX 75244
800-462-9273
www.komen.org
Nationwide series of runs/fitness walks (100+) benefiting breast cancer research, treatment, education, screening, outreach, and advocacy.

Terry Fox Run/Foundation
789 Don Mills Road, Suite 802
Toronto, ON M3C 1T5
416-962-7866
888-836-9786 (in Canada only)
www.terryfoxrun.org
Founded in memory of Terry Fox, who attempted to run across Canada after losing his leg to cancer. This Canadian-based organization raises money in local markets for cancer research through a series of over 5,600 road races around the world funded by the Four Seasons Hotel.

Us Too! International, Inc.
5003 Fairview Avenue
Downers Grove, IL 60515
630-795-1002
www.ustoo.org
Nationwide organization that offers fellowship, peer counseling, education about treatment options, and discussion of medical alternatives without bias for men and their families living with prostate cancer.

YMCA Encore Plus
Combination exercise and support programs for women with breast cancer conducted at YWCAs throughout the United States.

REGIONAL

The Brain Tumor Society
124 Watertown Street, Suite 3-H
Watertown, MA 02472
800-770-8287
617-924-9997
www.tbts.org
The Brain Tumor Society provides resources for patients, survivors, family, friends, and professionals.

Cancer Control Society
2043 North Berendo
Los Angeles, CA 90027
323-663-7801
www.cancercontrolsociety.com
One of the largest sources of the latest information on alternative medicine, including education, prevention, and control.

Team Survivor Los Angeles
1223 Wilshire Blvd, #570
Santa Monica, CA 90403-5400
310-829-7849
www.teamsurvivor-la.org
Provides exercise, health education, and support programs for women affected by cancer.

Wellness Community-West Los Angeles
2716 Ocean Park Blvd., Suite 1040
Santa Monica, CA 90405
310-314-2555
www.wellness-community.org
Helps people with cancer and their loved ones enhance their health and well-being by providing a professional program of emotional support, education, and hope.

INDEX

Abdominal crunches, 78, 95

Aerobic exercise, 4, 22, 29, 63
 brain tumor patients, 144–45
 breast cancer patients, 129–32
 cardiovascular training, 19, 83–84, 97,
   98
 colorectal cancer patients, 147–48
 heart rate training, 84
 intensity measurement, 77, 84
 leukemia/lymphoma/Hodgkin's disease
   patients, 143
 lung cancer patients, 139–40
 prostate cancer patients, 135–38
 walking, 67–68, 76, 77

American Cancer Society, 109, 173

American College of Sports Medicine,
   63, 83

American Council on Exercise, 83

American Dietetic Association, 162

Andersen, Barbara, 31

Anderson, David, 20

Annals of Behavioral Medicine, 61

Antioxidants, 106

Apple, baked, 115

Armstrong, Lance, 5–6, 25

Asian diet, 106

Atherosclerosis, and garlic, 122

Athletes Support Group for Cancer,
   14–16, 125, 150

Attitude and mindset, 23–27

Back extensions, 78–79

Berman, Jeff, 3, 21, 26, 34, 150
 cancer diagnosis of, 5–6, 8–11
 cancer-fighting approach of, 11–12,
   26–27, 166–68
 in chemotherapy, 12–13
 founding of FORCE program, 13–15
 in Three Miles of Men, 126

Beverages
 food choices/serving size, 113
 fruit smoothie, 117

Biceps curl, 64, 75, 81
    standing dumbbell, 94–95
Bicycling, 135
Bladder cancer, 99
Blair, Steve, 27–28
Blatnick, Jeff, 6, 149–50, 151
Blood clots, and garlic, 122
Blood count, benefits of exercise, 61,
    62
Blood thinner, ginkgo biloba as, 123
Bowel cancer, 60, 99
Brain tumor patients
    exercise and nutrition, 144–45
    treatment, 142
Breads
    English muffin pizza, 117
    fiber in, 105
    food choices/serving size, 110
    snacks, 117, 161
    waffles, 115
Breakfast, 105, 113–17, 160
Breast cancer, 31, 60, 99
    incidence of, 125
    Race for the Cure, 126–27
Breast cancer patients
    diet and nutrition, 129–32
    exercise modifications, 64–65, 127, 129
    exercise program, 127–28, 129–33
    and weight gain, 109
Breathing, deep, 30, 48–50, 58, 154–55
Burger, veggie/soy, 114
Buzzerio, John, 27, 28, 63, 156, 158

Calcium, 99
Calf raise, 73
Calf raise machine, standing, 88
Cancer
    benefits of diet and nutrition, 99–100,
        101, 103
    benefits of exercise, 1–2, 18–19
    as manageable chronic disease, 2–3
    and obesity, 109
    research on lifestyle benefits, 2, 3–4, 29,
        60–61, 99
    resources, 169–77
    and stress, 45–46
    support groups, 59
    treatment
        exercise during, 12–13, 19, 61–62
        herbal remedies as, 120–24
        and supplement claims, 118–119
    See also FORCE program
Cancer Care, 59, 170
Cardiovascular training, 19, 83–84, 97, 98
Cereals
    cold, 114
    fiber in, 105
    food choices/serving size, 110
    hot, 113
Chair squats, 72, 79
Change, stages of, 37–39, 100–101
Cheese
    cottage cheese and fruit platter, 115
    pizza, English muffin, 117
    See also Dairy products

Chemotherapy
exercise during, 12–13, 61–62
nutritional supplements during, 119
Chest press machine, seated, 93
Chicken
fajitas, 116
stir-fry, 114
wrap, 116
See also Poultry
Children with cancer
Kids Sports Day, 150–51
See also K-FORCE program
Chinese ginseng, 124
Chinese restaurants, 108, 115
Cisplatin, 124
Colon cancer, 109
Colorectal cancer patients, exercise and
nutrition for, 146–48
Condiments, 113
Conover, Mark, 6, 150
Contract, 40–41
Cooking methods, 102
Cool-down, 95–96
Cooper, Kenneth, 18–19
Cottage cheese and fruit platter, 115
Cousins, Norman, 26, 27
Cruciferous vegetables, 103
Curcumin, 123
Cytokines, 121

Dairy products
cottage cheese and fruit platter, 115

fat content of, 101
food choices/serving size, 111
pizza, English muffin, 117
Diabetes, 3
Diet and nutrition, 2, 22, 31–33, 100–101,
118
brain tumor patients, 144–45
breast cancer patients, 129–32
for children, 159–62
colorectal cancer patients, 147–48
fats in, 32, 101–3, 112
fiber in, 32, 105–6
food choices/serving size, 110–13
fruits and vegetables in, 32, 99, 103–4,
105, 110–11
leukemia/lymphoma/Hodgkin's disease
patients, 143
lung cancer patients, 139–40
meal plan, 7–day, 113–17
prostate cancer patients, 136–38
soy in, 32, 106–8, 111–12
supplements, 32, 118–19
See also specific foods
Dinner, 114–17, 160
Dumbbells, 68–69
biceps curl, standing, 94–95
shoulder press, standing, 92
triceps extension, standing one-arm, 95

Echinacea, 121
Eggs
food choices/serving size, 111

Eggs *(cont.)*
    omelet, egg white, 114
    scrambled, 116
Endorphins, 62
Esophagus cancer, 99
Essentials of Yoga, The (Sarley and Sarley),
        49
Exercise and cancer
    benefits during treatment, 12–13, 19,
        61–62
    preventive role of, 1–2, 60–61
    research on, 2, 3–4, 29, 60–61
Exercise/physical activity program, 22,
        27–29
    brain tumor patients, 144–45
    breast cancer patients, 64–65, 127–28,
        129–33
    for children, 156–59
    choice of exercise, 43–44
    colorectal cancer patients, 146–48
    cool-down, 95–96
    getting started, 41–42
    in gym setting. *See* Gyms and health clubs
    leukemia/lymphoma/Hodgkin's disease
        patients, 143
    lifestyle activities, 28, 68, 156–58
    lung cancer patients, 138–41
    maintenance, 96–98
    modifications/guidelines, 64–65
    overtraining, indicators of, 96
    with partner, 43, 65
    phase I, 66–76

phase II, 76–81
phase III, 81–96
prostate cancer patients, 134–38
at set times, 42–43, 65
10 percent rule, 65
training log, 42
types of movement, 63
warmups, 69, 86
See also Aerobic exercise; Resistance
        (weight) training

Fajitas, chicken, 116
Family
    modeling healthy behavior, 163–64
    protectiveness of, 26, 44
Fat, dietary, 32, 101–3, 112
Fatigue, benefits of exercise, 62
Fiber, dietary, 32, 105–6
Fight-or-flight response, 30, 46, 47
Fish
    fat in, 101
    food choices/serving size, 111
    salmon, honey mustard, 115
    sushi take-out, 117
    tuna pita, 116
    tuna salad, 113
Fish oil, 101
Fleegler, Fran, 2, 3, 34, 58, 60, 61, 168
Focus on Rehabilitation and Cancer
        Education. *See* FORCE program
Folic acid, 99
Food pyramid, 32

Foods. *See* Diet and nutrition; *specific foods*

FORCE program

attitude and mindset in, 23–27

balanced perspective of, 167

basic areas of, 22

for children. *See* K-FORCE program

and family involvement, 44

founding of, 6, 14–17

goals of, 2–3

media coverage of, 21

and oncologist-patient partnership,
    34–37

principles of, 4–5, 15–16

stages of change, 37–39

testimonials from graduates, 20–21

written agreement, 40–41

See also Diet and nutrition;
    Exercise/physical activity program;
    Stress management

Free radicals, 103

Friends in Deed, 15–16, 170

Fruits, 99

apple, baked, 115

and cottage cheese platter, 115

fiber in, 105

food choices/serving size, 111

phytochemicals in, 32, 103–4

smoothie, 117

snacks, 117, 161

Garlic, 103, 122

Gastric cancer, 124

Gilda's Club, 59, 174

Ginger, 122–23

Ginkgo Biloba, 123

Ginseng, 124

Grains, 105, 110

Green tea, 99, 113

Grieco, Regina, 157

Gyms and health clubs

cardiovascular training in, 83–84

personal trainers in, 82–83

resistance training in, 85–96

selecting, 81–82

Hamstring curl machine, prone, 87

Hanc, John, 13, 168

Hanson, Dave, 13

Harvard School of Public Health, 1–2

Health clubs. *See* Gyms and health clubs

Health magazine, 37–38

Heart rate

resting, 96, 98

target, 84

Heart rate monitor, 84

Hepatitis, 3

Herbal remedies, 32, 120–24

Hip-extension machine, 45–degree, 91

Hodgkin's disease patients, 149–50

children, 163–64

exercise and nutrition for, 141, 143

Hugs, daily, 58

Humor, 26–27

Hypertension, 3

Imagination scrapbook exercise, 153–54

Immune system

and echinacea, 121

and garlic, 122

and stress, 45

Indoles, 103

Insomnia, benefits of exercise, 62

Interferon, 121

Interleukins, 121

International Health Racquet and

Sportsclub Association, 82

Joint flexibility, benefits of exercise, 62

Kalman, Douglas S., 32, 119, 120

Kennedy, Deborah, 162

K-FORCE program

diet and nutrition, 159–62

parental role in, 163–65

philosophy of, 151–53

physical activity, 156–58

strength training, 158–59

stress management, 153–56

Kidney cancer, 109

Kid Sports Day, 150–51

Knee hugs, double, 71, 77

Komen (Susan G.) Breast Cancer

Foundation, 126, 174

Ladas, Elena, 162

Lebow, Fred, 13–15, 16

Lecithin, 106

Leg press machine, horizontal, 86

Legumes, fiber in, 105

Leukemia patients, 6, 9

exercise and nutrition for, 141, 143

Life force, essential, 49

Lifestyle activities, 28, 68, 156–58

Lifestyle treatments. *See* Diet and

nutrition; Exercise/physical

activity program; Stress

management

Liquori, Marty, 6

Low-fat diet, 32, 99, 102–3

Lowry, Genevieve, 151, 154

Lunch, 113–17, 160

Lung cancer patients, exercise and

nutrition for, 138–41

Lunges, 79

split, 74

Lycopene, 99, 103

Lymphoma patients, exercise and

nutrition for, 141–42, 143

Mastectomy/lumpectomy, exercise and

nutrition, 64, 130–32

Meal plan, 7-day, 113–17

Meat

cooking methods, 102

fat content of, 101, 102

food choices/serving size, 111

Medicine & Science in Sports & Exercise,

83

Meditation, 30, 54–56

Memorial Sloan-Kettering Cancer Center, 150, 166

Mental imagery, 52–54, 153–54

Milk

    food choices/serving size, 111

    soy milk, 106–7, 111

Miso soup, 107

Monounsaturated fat, 101

Mood, benefits of exercise, 62

Morgan, Barbara, 21

Mt. Sinai Wellness Program, 17

Muscle relaxation, progressive (PMR), 50–52, 154

Muscle strength, benefits of exercise, 62

National Cancer Institute, 2

National Strength and Conditioning Association, 83

Negative emotions, 23

Neporent, Liz, 74

Neuropathy, 62

New England Journal of Medicine, 60–61

New York City Marathon, 13–14, 16

New York Road Runners Club, 13, 14–15

Nutrition. *See* Diet and nutrition

Nutritional counseling, 22

Nutritional supplements, 32, 118–19

Nye, Bill, 17

Obesity, 109

Oils, 101, 102, 112

Omega-3 fatty acids, 101, 102

Omega-6 fatty acids, 101, 102

Omelet, egg white, 114

Oncologists, 3, 20, 34–37

Organosulfur compounds, 103

Ovarian cancer, 124

Overtraining, indicators of, 96

Pasta, 105, 110, 160

    primavera, 116

Patton approach, 23

Peale, Norman Vincent, 24

Personal trainer, 82–83

Phenols, 123

Physical activity. *See* Exercise/physical activity program

Physicians. *See* Oncologists

Phytic acid, 106

Phytochemicals, 32, 103–4, 106

Phytoestrogens, 32

Pizza, 160

    English muffin, 117

Platelet counts, benefits of exercise, 62

Play activities, for children, 156–58

Pogran, Arthur, 21

Polyunsaturated fat, 101

Positive thinking, 24

Potato coins, 114

Poultry

    chicken fajitas, 116

    chicken stir-fry, 114

    chicken wrap, 116

    cooking methods, 102

Poultry *(cont.)*
  fat content of, 101, 102
  food choices/serving size, 111
  turkey and (almost) all the fixins, 115
  turkey sandwich, 114
Powers, Nancy, 150
Prana concept, 49
Preventive medicine, 1–2, 18–19
Prochaska, James, 37–38
Progressive muscle relaxation (PMR),
  50–52
Prostate cancer, 60, 99
Prostate cancer patients
  and bicycling, 135
  diet and nutrition, 136–38
  exercise modifications, 134, 136
  exercise program, 134–38
  organizations and activism, 128,
  133–34
Protectiveness, family, 26, 44
Pull-down machine, seated cable lat, 90
Push-ups, modified, 81, 158

Race for the Cure, 126–27
Raphael, Bruce, 9, 10, 11, 12
Relaxation techniques, 4, 16, 30
  for children, 154
  meditation, 54–56
  progressive muscle relaxation (PMR),
  50– 52
Resistance (weight) training, 4, 22, 29, 63
  brain tumor patients, 144–45

breast cancer patients, 64–65, 127–28,
  129–33
for children, 158–59
colorectal cancer patients, 147–48
with dumbbells. *See* Dumbbells
elastic tubing workouts, 127–28
leukemia/lymphoma/Hodgkin's disease
  patients, 143
for lung cancer patients, 139–40
maintenance workouts, 97–98
with personal trainer, 82–83
phase I exercises, 70–76
phase II exercises, 77–81
phase III exercises, 83–96
prostate cancer patients, 134–35,
  136–38
Restaurants
  soy foods in, 107–8
  take-out, 115, 117
Rheumatism, postchemotherapy, 62
Rice, 105, 110
Rosenhagen, Bette Jean, 30, 49, 50
Row exercise, one arm bent over, 80
Row machine, seated, 89

Salads, 116
  and soup lunch, 115
  tuna, 113, 160
Salmon, honey mustard, 115
Salomon, Heather, 32, 101, 104, 159,
  166
Sandwiches, 160

chicken wrap, 116

tuna pita, 116

turkey, 114

Saponin, 106

Sarley, Dinabandhu and Ila, 49

Saturated fat, 101

Selenium, 99

Self-Healing, 21

Shaffer, Richard, 40

Shoulder press, 65, 80

standing dumbbell, 92

Siberian ginseng, 124

Snacks, 112, 117, 160, 161

Social support, 58–59

Soup

miso, 107

and salad lunch, 115

Soy

burger, 114

food choices/serving size, 106–8, 111–12

phytochemicals in, 32, 106

Soy milk, 106–7, 111

Soy protein, powdered/textured, 107, 111

Spirituality, 58

Split lunges, 74

Step-ups, 158–59

Strength training. *See* Resistance (weight) training

Stress

and cancer, 45–46

defined, 30

positive and negative, 46–47

Stress management, 2, 5, 16, 22, 30–31, 47–48

at bedtime, 57

breathing, deep, 30, 48–50, 58

for children, 153–56

meditation, 30, 54–56

mental imagery/visualization, 30, 52–54, 153–54

muscle relaxation, progressive (PMR), 50–52

and social support, 58–59

and spirituality, 58

and touching, 58

Two-Minute Drill, 57–58

Stress test, 84

Supplements, 32, 118–19

Support groups, 59

Surgeon General, *Report on Exercise and Physical Activity,* 27–28, 60

Susan G. Komen Breast Cancer Foundation, 126, 174

Sushi take-out, 117

Tacos, 160

Tea, 113

Tempeh, 107, 111

Three Miles of Men, 126

Tofu, 107, 108, 111, 115

Tomatoes, 99, 103

Touch, 58

Trans-fatty acids, 101

Triceps extensions, 64, 76, 81

   standing one-arm dumbbell, 95

Truman, Harry S., 67

Tube workouts, 127–28

Tumor necrosis factor, 121

Tuna

   pita, 116

   salad, 113, 160

Turkey

   and (almost) all the fixins, 115

   sandwich, 114

   See also Poultry

Unsaturated fat, 101

Urine, color of, 108

Us Too!, 128, 134, 176

Uterine cancer, 109

Vegetables, 99

   fiber in, 105

   food choices/serving size, 110

   pasta primavera, 116

   phytochemicals in, 32, 103–4

   pizza, English muffin, 117

   potato coins, 114

   snacks, 117, 161

Veggie burger, 114

Visualization, 30, 52–54, 153–54

Vitamin A, 99, 103

Vitamin C, 99, 103

Vitamin D, 99

Vitamin E, 99

Volleyball, Wall, 64, 70–71

Waffles, 115

Walking, 67–68, 76, 77

Walking shoes, 67–68

Wall volleyball, 64, 70–71

Warmups, 69, 86

Water consumption

   and body's requirements, 108

   during exercise, 65, 98, 156

Weight gain, 109

Weight training. *See* Resistance (weight)

   training

Weil, Andrew, 21, 48–49

Wellness Community, 59

Yoga, breathing in, 49

Zale Foundation, 17

ABOUT THE AUTHORS

JEFF BERMAN is a cancer survivor who now runs FORCE (Focus on Rehabilitation and Cancer Education) full-time. He worked with the legendary founder of the New York Road Runners Club, Fred Lebow, to establish the first exercise support group for people with cancer, which became the FORCE program five years later. He has established support programs at Memorial Sloan-Kettering Cancer Center and has been awarded grants to spread the word about FORCE's effectiveness and to establish more branches.

FRAN FLEEGLER, M.D., was educated at the University of Pittsburgh medical school and the University of Pennsylvania, where she served as a clinical associate professor in the medical school. She is a member of the American Society of Clinical Oncology and the American College of Sports Medicine, and serves as a clinical adviser for the American Running Association. Dr. Fleegler, who is herself a competitive distance runner, lives in Boulder, Colorado, where she is affiliated with Rocky Mountain Cancer Center.

JOHN HANC is a writer specializing in active sports and fitness. A columnist and contributing writer to *Newsday* and a frequent contributor to *Runner's World* magazine, Hanc has written four previous books, including *The Essential Runner* and *Running for Dummies*, which he coauthored with the late Florence Griffith Joyner.